DR. PETER HOFMANN

DENTISTRY

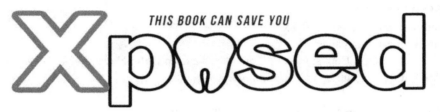

THIS BOOK CAN SAVE YOU

Protecting You, Your Smile, and Your Wallet

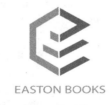

EASTON BOOKS

— Everyone Has A Story —

DENTISTRY XPOSED

Protecting You, Your Smile, and Your Wallet

Author: Dr. Peter Hofmann, DDS
© Copyright Dr. Peter Hofmann DDS, All Rights Reserved Media and Press Contact: http://www.Dentistryxposed.com

Paperback: 129 pages
Language: English
ISBN-13: 978-1-0878-0366-1

ASIN: B081VV84FD
Product Dimensions: 6 x 0.3 x 9 inches
Print Length: 145 pages
Publisher: Easton Books; First Edition   **Publication Date:** November 4, 2019
Distribution: Ingram Spark   **Language:** English

Library of Congress Registration Number: TX 8-840-661

NOTICE

This book is intended as a reference for you to research topics and interact with professionals and others. This is not a medical manual nor a cure-all. To the fullest extent of the law, no responsibility is assumed by Easton Books or the author for any injury and/or damage to persons or property as a matter of products liability, negligence, or ideas contained in the material herein. The anecdotal accounts are true and notable, and the author does not claim to be the final authority. The author advises patients to seek second opinions. He fully acknowledges the integrity of American dentistry, all affiliated officials, and the community of healthcare providers.

Acknowledgment

Rebecca Nietert at Easton-Books, who taught the intricacies of book publishing and helped shape the design of this book.

Angie McCutcheon and Diane Jay who were an inspiration & generous in their willingness to work alongside me.

Dedication

Dr. Hofmann dedicates this book to all his wonderful patients that inspired him to change and create a better solution.

CONTENTS

ANSWERS AND INFORMATION

Answers to Help You, Your Wallet, and Those You Love:

- A Substance that is both cheap and sweet yet can stop bad bacteria.
- Amazing new material removes decay without a needle or drill.

Information that Exposes Myths, Lies, and Falsehoods:

1. -Why is dentistry expensive & how to make good treatment decisions?
-Why are sugars & acids like Apple Cider Vinegar bad for my teeth?
-How is the mouth related to the 3 Most Common Causes of Death?

2. -Is Big Pharma manufacturing disease with drugs that cause dry mouth?
-What are some of the biggest scams in dentistry and how to avoid them?
-How to recognize signs of Sleep Apnea in your children & others.
-Why are the new space-age Zirconia crowns so effective for teeth?

3. -24 Myths in the Mouth, and 30 Doc, I did not know that, answers.
-Does alcohol in Listerine or in alcoholic beverages cause cancer?
-How can this book guarantee you will save a lot of money, time and pain?

4. -Is a dry cough related to sleep disorders & is there a simple cure?
-Is there a connection between the mouth and cancer of the pancreas?
-What are the simple and almost FREE ways to protect teeth and gums?
-What are AGE's and acrylates, & how and why can they be deadly?

CHAPTER ONE
Introduction
Finding Health

Understand that your Good Health begins with the mouth and what happens there affects your whole body and quality of life. The mouth is your *signature organ* which can play out with a smile, kiss, or a beautiful sound. It serves to warn us of stress, immune responses, diseases and vitamin deficiencies. Your mouth and smile can help you achieve your dreams. As Louis Armstrong so beautifully sang, "When You're Smiling the Whole World Smiles with You."

With forty-three years of experience as an urban and wilderness dentist, author and inventor Dr. Hofmann is committed to helping you. Some answers will be as simple as having a high spot on a tooth adjusted, using a simple and safe spray to stop a dry hacking cough, or drinking the table water at your meal to rinse away food debris. He will inform you about many amazing products including a "wonder molecule" that prevents tooth decay and protects the mucosal linings from head to colon, or a new discovery that destroys tooth decay without a needle or drill. His observations will save you money and your health.

This information is for everyone including those who have little or no understanding of their mouth. For example, a handicapped patient found it convenient to go to a dentist within walking distance of his apartment. He was told he needed extensive and very expensive gum surgery along with a series of deep cleanings. In a state of panic, he made an appointment to see Dr. Hofmann. Over many years the patient had eroded his teeth by over-brushing. Although his x-rays showed large ghost-like spots in those areas, this type of tooth erosion is not a disease and does not require surgery nor a deep cleaning! The deep cleaning or surgery would have harmed his healthy pink gum tissue. He was extremely grateful to hear the truth and thus save thousands of dollars.

At key points in this book, the author will present a question or issue without providing direct answers. This should inspire you to think so you can come to your own conclusion while avoiding libelous judgments. Eventually logic and common-sense will shape a good answer. An example is evidence showing "manufactured disease" in the mouth. Over 500 medications produced by the drug industry causes dry mouth which leads to tooth decay or periodontal disease. Research shows that this will feed bad bacteria and toxins or enzymes into the blood stream. These in turn can cause heart disease, joint inflammation, pancreatitis and other disorders. A dry mouth also allows bacterial plaques to form around teeth and to be inhaled causing pneumonia. It is a death trap waiting to happen to those who are aging, incapacitated, or bedridden. Pneumonia is the #1 cause of death.

Some data might be contested by invested corporations or interest groups. Dr. Hofmann will leave the logical conclusions up to you and hopes that you will be both informed and inspired. Try not to self-diagnose nor treat any serious condition on your own. If some words or terms are difficult, go to Chapter12 which will explain them. This knowledge will help you research any topic in more depth.

The information presented will save you both time and money. It may also rescue a life. Just observing how a person breathes may end up saving them! A nasal sound is evidence of potential sleep apnea which if untreated can lead to a heart attack or other serious consequences. Sleep apnea can cause severe stress to the pancreas, brain and other organs and increase the chance for cancer or strokes. It can harm people of every age. An alarm concerning this danger needs to be sounded.

This book will also address many of the myths, falsehoods and serious deceptions on the trail to the truth. Some are anecdotal accounts with important data that will help you and those you love to avoid many pitfalls along the way to good health. In order to insure a balanced and honest viewpoint, *Dr. Hofmann has been very careful not to accept money from any company.* However, he will share information on certain products that have proven themselves effective in preventing or healing disease. Some of the important ones are backed up by decades of good research.

One pitfall that will surprise readers is the Apple Cider Vinegar craze which promotes itself as a cure-all for dieting and healing for everything from acid reflux to respiratory issues. A recent promotion claimed "1000 tried-and-true remedies" which will heal you. The promoters fail to mention when you habitually sip a diluted vinegar-acid it can cause major tooth decay. As you make important choices remember those "natural home remedies" often do not list critical contraindications or warnings.

Our lives are already too full of cravings and desires which have stoked addictions and other bad choices. These include smoking, e-cigs, vaping, marijuana, opioids and the ever-growing sugar and snack food habits, all of which are increasing in the youth. Hopefully this book will help you overcome those pitfalls so that you can move forward to experience relief and healing. Your life should not be a measure of lost time, but of good safe choices and a transformation that will allow you to become a healthier and better person.

Dentistry is committed to preventive care and to treating pain with the least amount of discomfort. If preventive dentistry has not been a big part of your dental health, this book will be of special importance, as it shows you concepts which will improve your technique. If you had a painful experience going to the dentist, information revealed will give you renewed confidence. And note, most dentists are honest and hardworking, very knowledgeable and dedicated to helping you deal with fear or pain in a comfortable way. Dr. Hofmann desires to improve dentistry throughout the world by educating and forewarning the reader about conditions and issues few have known about or understood. He invites you to join him on this journey of transformation.

He intends to be an advocate for those who cannot afford the cost of treatment in the modern dental office and believes the information in this book will change the lives of many who read it. For instance, there are many simple and effective ways to prevent and control both tooth decay and gum disease that most people do not know about. Much of this information has not been shared nor is being taught to patients.

Many people, including doctors, do not know that there is a simple food medicine that inactivates bad bacteria in the mouth, ears, nose, throat and gut! It will prevent tooth decay and can cure sinusitis, an earache or a hacking cough as it did for Dr. Hofmann. Chapters such as "WOW 2 WHOA," "DOC, I Did Not Know That," and "Myth Busting," will reveal stunning information that can help you make decisions which will positively affect your health and wallet. This information is based on many research studies.

As you read on, each chapter will have special ALERTS to point you to important data or observations. They will be accented with italics or statements like, "it may surprise you to know." For instance, it may surprise you to know that using two toothbrushes to allow each to dry out will help prevent bacterial recontamination.

Did you know teeth comprise only 20% of the mouth? The other 80% is soft tissue, tongue and mucosa, all of which are moistened by an important saliva people take for granted? Knowing the value of your saliva should motivate you to take steps to nurture and preserve it. Evidence shows that dry mouth weakens saliva and will lead to tooth decay and gum disease that can then hurt your heart. Drugs that affect saliva include ibuprofen, antihistamines, opioids, and diuretics. Habits such as smoking or consuming soft drinks will have a bad impact on saliva. Many of us have a level of addictive behavior or habit that affects our health. This book will help make it clear why and how they are harmful, so that you can then take the right counter measures.

There are other forces in your mouth which can sabotage both your health and your wallet. For instance, when you put off seeing a dentist after a crown falls off, natural shifting will occur in surrounding teeth which can cost you hundreds of dollars to correct. Your restoration will no longer fit, and a new crown may have to be made. Or if you fail to wear your new partial denture, teeth will move and the denture will no longer fit. As you continue reading take notes and if the book does not save you money you can have your money back.

Some products like toothbrushes are engineered for fashion and to fool you. Have you noticed that soft toothbrushes do not feel soft? Bristles are placed tightly together in pointed tufts that create two problems. One is that bacterial plaque or colonies are easily preserved in those tight places. If bristles are placed further apart air dries and kills the bacteria. A tuft is also more abrasive and destructive to thin tissue and weak dentin. This aggregation of bristles creates a hard pointed nob. The solution is simple: just use tufts with fewer bristles that will allow more bending and more air flow. This may not seem "sexy" to the manufacturers who seem intent on creating a new colorful design every year!

This book is unique for it is designed to get your attention and equip you to be able to talk to your dentist concerning your oral health care needs. Therefore, share it with your family, friends, strangers, and of course your dentist. Each chapter has powerful information that will inform even the highly educated. We have all been brainwashed to some extent by the sugar industry, media ads, and by our personal experiences or exposure to medicine and dentistry. We cannot trust commercials to keep ourselves or our kids healthy. The worse thing we can do is reward children with sugar or sweet snacks when they act up, have emotional needs, or are just demanding. Snack foods can act as sugar on steroids as they will use up the resources needed for digestion and act as a very sticky plaque in the mouth.

Keep an open perspective and use Internet search engines to find specific information that will help you better understand any topic discussed in this book. Dr. Peter Hofmann thanks you for buying the book, studying and sharing the information presented. He appreciates your observations, responses or reviews and hopes that you will help support and spread this grass-roots effort to wake people up to the truth related to dentistry and healthcare - so that lives can be saved.

CHAPTER TWO
<u>The Good - The Wise</u>
The Bad, and The Ugly

Knowledge can guide us to excellent health through both prevention and intervention. Knowledge alone, however, is often not enough. Motivation to act and follow through with good habits requires a little risk taking. To achieve change you may have to try something that runs counter to your thinking. For instance, try the super-soft Korean packet of four super-soft toothbrushes. You will be amazed how well they clean and last. They will not irritate and erode fragile bone and gums like harder toothbrushes.

More truth will be uncovered as this book shines a light on exciting oral care concepts, good and bad dental products, ugly scams, falsehoods and myths, and observations that will warn you before disease or pain sets in. Unfortunately, the exposing of truth will step on some feet, such as some Wall Street companies and those who preach with the profit motive, promoting Hollywood hyper-whites and speedy treatments with titles like *How to make a Million Quickly* or *Spend Less Time & Make More Money!*

Quality time is what every patient needs with his or her dentist. The patient should be made aware of their condition, the cost and length of treatment, and all options available. It is important that the dentist warns you of any consequences or emergencies which might arise. After all, your mouth is a unique organ which requires attention as you eat, drink, and breathe.

Chewing is the ultimate "stress test" to determine how effective a restoration will be. You deserve fillings and other solutions that stand the test of time. In turn it is your responsibility explore the good techniques and concepts taught in this book and then transform any bad habits into good ones.

To eat and drink healthy means to avoid excess sugar, empty calories such as processed carbohydrates and acidic foods and drinks. Unfortunately, most things we like are acidic, sweet, or quick and easy to eat. So, what is the answer? A great solution is to drink plenty of water and eat only when you are hungry. If you drink wine, fruit juices, soft drinks, or use apple cider vinegar, rinse with water afterwards and swallow. If possible, drink with a straw. When you snack rinse with water and skip those empty calories. They are like sugar to the body.

Search out foods that have more fiber such as bran or seeded bread, and raw or steamed vegetables. Experiment by eating salads with nuts, fruit, dried cranberries, goat cheese, or a hard-boiled egg. Eat cauliflower and fruits like strawberries or plums which have natural xylitol. These foods make good snacks as xylitol works to inactivate cavity forming bacteria in your mouth. The xylitol protects the saliva, the microbiome of your gut and your nasopharyngeal passages from dangerous bacteria and yeast.

Mouth malodor or Halitosis by itself can be a big turn-off to social acceptance and good communication. This seems like a little problem, but it can be a sign of a much bigger issue. Brushing your tongue, teeth, and gums with a super-soft toothbrush will help. Seeing your dentist for a regular checkup and using antiseptic mouth rinses helps. Use warm water with a touch of salt or chlorine dioxide mouth rinse to neutralize sulfurous odors. Chlorine dioxide has been shown to be very effective against Sulphur compounds and related bacteria that cause malodor. If a dry mouth is causing odors use xylitol to increase your salivary flow.

Cutting down on those manufactured snacks or empty calories will also protect your teeth by letting your saliva recuperate from acids. In following chapters, we will learn how important your saliva is and how helpful it is to use xylitol mints or chewing gum to neutralize acids. Toothpaste and mouth rinses with added zinc protect teeth and help to counter bad breath, especially in combination with activated chlorine dioxide rinses. Mouth odors can also come from a dry mouth and from infections in gums and within deep decay.

Scattered throughout the book are examples of good decisions and bad mistakes one can make concerning the care and use of the mouth. Some of those mistakes are due to popular myths and bad media-medicine. Others may be due to the confusing science of dentistry. Most professions do not have so many strange words, double meanings, and the weird gadgets associated with them.

Dr. Hofmann's personal experiences will challenge you to make wise decisions concerning your preventive care. Two widely advertised examples of potentially bad media-medicine are apple cider vinegar and extensive nasal flushes that wipe away good mucosa. We will discuss these in later chapters.

Hopefully this book will become a go-to reference resource you will share with your family, friends, co-workers and acquaintances. Get your highlighter out and take notes. Explore the Chapter on Terminology as you go along. All words are printed in this *"script format"* are defined and explained there.

Use caution if you are using baking soda or hydrogen peroxide to clean or disinfect your teeth. Ironically some people use these in sensitive areas thinking they will heal tissue. The truth is just the opposite. They destroy the microbiome that protects the teeth and gums. Do not use this combination for receding or eroded gums or bone. Both baking soda and salt crystals are too abrasive. Many modern toothpastes have rounded micro-particles of sodium bicarbonate, calcium carbonate or other semi-abrasives that clean safely and effectively when used with a good super-soft toothbrush. If you are very careful in areas of recession, you may avoid the need for surgery.

Another simple solution that has surprised many of Dr. Hofmann's patients is how effective and durable his specially engineered super-soft brushes are. Some people tend to reject the super soft concept because of false thinking. They do not realize that a super-soft bristle is much kinder to tissue as it reaches around into very tight areas. Amazingly, it cleans better and does not wear down quickly. The new tougher design keeps the bristles sterile as room air circulates easily around each bristle keeping them dry and preventing cross-contamination from bacteria.

In this 21st Century, dentists should be producing better, safer, and more ethical dentistry - Right? Our oral health should be better than in the 50's, and we should all have beautiful smiles. Well, we know this is not always true! Advanced dentistry has given us a revolutionary crown material that is both tooth-colored and super-strong. And if you lose all your teeth, the amazing "All-on-4 implant" can solve the problem. An unattractive smile or a bad bite can be reshaped with clear aligners or fast braces. The computerized digital x-ray allows the patient to see their teeth on a big screen quickly and uses six times less radiation. Regenerative surgeries grow new bone and tissue where bone has shrunk away after a tooth has been pulled. This was not thought possible a generation ago.

So, what is the problem? One obvious answer is that math and science do not resolve the question of cost, fear, and moral or ethical issues. These ethical issues will eventually lead us to an ugly aspect of dentistry. This discussion and revelation should guide you as you chose dental treatment in the future. It should motivate you get a second opinion when something seems unusual or beyond your expectations and past experiences. For instance, there seems to be a propensity in certain dental practices to diagnosis healthy gums as needing the much more expensive deep cleaning. This is a very profitable scam for any dental office. If your gums are healthy, a deep cleaning can hurt you. So get a second opinion and report the situation to a dental society.

Added to this equation are the bad habits and bad practices that one can fall into. Some of these untamed factors affect both the good patient and the good dentist. We will see how sharply and deeply they cut into both our wallets and our joy. And as we do this, realize that the sugar industry is not your friend; they are devoted to keeping you addicted to sugar. They are not about to help you or anyone else discover safer solutions. Traditional sugar and sugar products feed the diabetes epidemic, tooth decay and the pervasive periodontal disease which science proves is linked to heart disease. Sugar has also been blamed for increasing the risk of Candida infections, auto immune disease, some mental conditions, diabetes, pancreatitis, and both pancreatic and colon cancer.

The effects of sugar is a huge burden on healthcare in all nations, with estimates of cost totally a trillion dollars a year! The healthcare cost of sugar in America in 2017 was 172 billion. The book *Soda Politics, Taking on Big Soda,* estimates that Coca Cola will spend 12 billion marketing its drinks in Africa and that Pepsi will spend 5 billion in India. Candies are another big threat to the health of poor kids all over this earth. The IADR (International & American Associations of Dental Research) estimates that in 2015 the world spent $442 billion treating just dental diseases! By 2020 it may double.

Health Organizations recognize the beneficial effects of anti-bacterial xylitol. Why is our FDA so quiet? Has the sugar cartel managed to suppress the truth about the natural preventive effects of this acid-fighting sugar? Xylitol is the best answer to counter worsening health conditions of people around the world and to lower the high cost of healthcare. Countering this is the sugar industry with its artificial sweeteners and fad sugars that destroy tissues, teeth and organs. In following chapters we will see how concentrated sugars like High Fructose Corn Syrup have become an even greater threat to health.

CHAPTER THREE

What Can Go Wrong?

Facts & Confessions

Dr. Hofmann is what one would call a traditional dentist and recognizes that his parent's world of medicine was in many ways more primitive, painful, and slower. His uncle who was an excellent dentist, used a belt-driven *handpiece* which smelled of smoke and burning oil as it spun around polishing teeth. Gold and mercury amalgams were the favored materials for crowns and fillings. The barber-like pump-chairs and spittoons with swirling water added to the noise and anxiety.

Dentists were exposed to mercury, heavy particles in the air, loud noise, radiation, back and neck strain, and a lot of bacterial contamination. When drilling teeth dentists did not wear masks nor gloves! This may be why dentistry was known to have the highest suicide and mortality rate. This is no longer true. Dentistry is now much safer. Despite being exposed to many of these dangers a good part of the boomer generation has enjoyed long lifespans.

Imagine what has happened in just 50 years! Now that implants are so successful, modern dentistry has in many ways been transformed beyond the tooth-centered concepts of saving and restoring weak teeth to the present concept of focusing on ideal Implant size, position, and function while creating the perfect smile and bite. Now a highlighted solution for major decay, tooth fracture, periodontal disease, or chewing failure is the tooth implant and not the root canal, tooth-supported bridge, or partial-denture.

The science of *Implantology* has motivated the use and development of ceramic Zirconia crowns, resin cements, sinus lift surgeries, and bone regeneration. These new ceramic crowns are beautiful in color, do not erode opposing teeth like the once popular porcelain crowns did, and are so strong a hammer cannot break them.

Do not be confused by the word "ceramic;" it is not at all related to pottery. These tooth-colored crowns are a high-tech metal-ceramic engineered by the Space Shuttle   project. This is a perfect combination for the longer lasting human

9

life in pursuit of happiness. Indeed, we are living in the golden age of dentistry. The picture below compares the inferior porcelain crown to the Zirconia ceramic crown.

Fig. 1

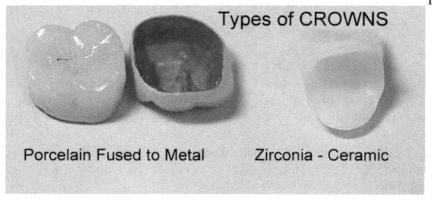

Types of CROWNS

Porcelain Fused to Metal   Zirconia - Ceramic

What could possibly go wrong? To most of us who have good teeth and healthy gums, it all seems OK! However, are you ready to handle the broken tooth or a deep pain emergency? Has the stress of life affected your mouth? People who experience tooth erosion, or worn out teeth from grinding, or the pervasive receding of gums know how unattractive and sensitive it can be. Did you know there is a simple effective way to rid yourself of sensitivity? Are you prepared for the shock of an expensive deep cleaning, periodontal "gum surgery" or a full reconstruction of your entire mouth due to excessive wear on chewing surfaces? Is your beautiful white smile being chipped away? Are you developing facial wrinkles because your bite is collapsing?

Are you tired during the day and wake up in the middle of the night sweating or in a panic? Has anyone suggested a sleep therapy study? Are you trying to save a tooth the dentist has suggested you pull? Are you aware that a chronic infection around your tooth can hurt your heart? Are you introducing dangerous bacteria into your mouth from dirty hands or from your pet or sex partners? Do you know others who need help in these areas?

The point of this book is not to scare you but to educate you so you can recognize issues or bad habits before they put your health and life at risk. With this knowledge you can educate others and communicate better with your hygienist or dentist. Dr. Hofmann confesses, "I am thankful, to have had my own personal health and dental problems. This has helped me to understand many of the issues and problems patients have. As a child

I loved sugar and remember eating butter and sugar on white bread. Luckily, I grew up with fluoridated water or I would not have the teeth I have. However, that sugar habit did feed colonies of Strep in my mouth that would often multiply and cause strep throat."

Many years ago Dr. Hofmann was shown a simple spray on solution that can conquer Strep bacterium. It can replace the need for antibiotics. Taking penicillin over-and-over again can develop a resistant form of the bacteria. And penicillin takes a least 24-48 hours to be absorbed in the intestinal lining. It must then pass through the blood stream to reach the head and neck. A simple and more effective way is to use xylitol as a spray to inactivate the Strep directly. This is just one of many positive health effects that xylitol can do for you! This concept also protects the microbiome in the mouth and gut from antibiotics. Dr. Hofmann did not learn this from the media nor the health community. The health system seems to have a large blind spot to some very good preventive concepts that are accepted by other nations. Hopefully you will let this book open your eyes.

Some of you have had the experience of biting an olive or cherry pit and then feeling a crunch which hopefully was the seed cracking and not your tooth. In Dr. Hofmann's case it was both, but the tooth did not break apart. What happened is very common. A craze-line was formed which would hurt on occasion on chewing. He thought that it was an upper tooth but while on a trip a big part of his lower molar cracked off and the pain went away. He had been a victim of referred pain which can cause people to seek treatment on the wrong tooth. Information like this should help you to make good decisions that will save you money and keep you from more pain.

"I have a small family practice in a very big city which could allow for a certain amount of bias on my part," explains Dr. Hofmann. "A patient or dentist in a big city may face a different set of challenges and circumstances than a person in a small town. My location for instance has many large managed care practices that promoted their brands with major TV ads. My area also has a number of solo-practices that do heavy advertising online."

Statistics indicate most dental practices today are either corporately owned, a group practice, or belong to a managed care network. Despite their corporate connections many of these practices create an image of being a simple private practice. Most are not traditional solo practices where you can be certain to see the same dentist each time you visit. What works in a small practice may not work as well in these large networks, as they often depend on large staffs of hygienists, managers, dentists, and assistants.

You should have a one-to-one interaction with your dentist so you can learn to deal effectively with your special preventive needs and challenges. With a mirror in-hand and digital x-rays to illustrate the problems, you will better understand the condition in your mouth so that you are able to comprehend the many options and treatment choices available.

A new patient who had been having her teeth cleaned in another office for many years had many problems that she was not aware of. Dr. Hofmann and his hygienist counted over a dozen different issues that needed her attention including excessive wear on her occlusion, a crossbite, a heavily discolored craze line, and recession that might eventually need surgery. It is important that patients are reminded of untreated problems each time they return for a recall cleaning. Dr. Hofmann emphasizes repetition and visual reinforcement of information since people often do not hear nor comprehend instructions the first time.

This is one more reason why the book is called Dentistry Xposed. The more we are exposed to good teaching and the good results which follow, the quicker we will adapt our lifestyle to safe and healthy habits. Otherwise chronic conditions such as periodontal disease and tooth erosion can accelerate the need for surgery or a major over-haul of the chewing surfaces. The dental chair is the perfect place to educate the patient and help him or her with nutrition and preventive techniques.

Dr. Hofmann has practiced dentistry for 43 years, providing care in Dallas. He has done this after completing hundreds of hours of continuing education and with a degree from the dental school which *"U.S. News & World Report"* declared the #1 dental school in the U.S. for each year over a ten-year time span. He has had to confront many important issues, one of which is the use of amalgam fillings. He believes patients are better off not removing old metal fillings that are in good shape! These fillings are much stronger than white fillings and the bigger ones can resist heavy chewing forces much better than white fillings. Depending on location these metal alloys can last 2 to 5 times longer. Some last a lifetime.

Would you rather keep an old metal filling for 40-50 years as he has or find yourself having to repair or replace white fillings in just a few years; especially if they are large or medium fillings? This can also lead to expensive crown restorations. Just flossing and chewing can erode the white fillings located between back teeth. This can open gaps in the contact areas between teeth which in turn will create major food traps that can lead to periodontal disease and bone loss.

Any white filling which spans over one-third the width of a tooth is weak and can erode as the upper cusp digs into it over-and-over again. Some of these white fillings incorporate the plastic BPA which will be swallowed as it is eroded away. White fillings work perfectly well on front teeth and can last longer but everyone needs to be aware that chewing with heavy pressure or tearing plastic wrappings with the front teeth can dislodge or break these fillings. Likewise, those who grind or grit their teeth need to take special precautions. Those who grind should wear a hard night-time mouth guard and daytime clinchers should wear a soft day-guard that does not affect speech. The hard surface allows for sliding movements of the jaw whereas the soft lets the patient clinch softly.

Those who grind in their sleep will often show extensive wear on their teeth. One clear sign of wear is short front teeth that have been worn down. As large or medium white fillings on back teeth wear down the front teeth will grind against each other at a faster rate. Look at a door hinge: a small movement near the hinge causes a much greater movement near the door handle. The area next to the hinge may close an inch while the door-handle moves a foot. The jaw works in the same fashion; as you wear down a millimeter in the back, you can double or triple wear on front teeth.

Healthy teeth can be easily worn down by abrasive actions of porcelain crowns. This loss will allow greater wear to all the remaining teeth. The illustration below shows how a little wear on back teeth results in much greater wear in the front anterior teeth. The back second molars in gray have lost one millimeter of enamel while the front incisors have lost more due to grinding:

Fig. 2 - The black area marks where grinding has eroded enamel away:

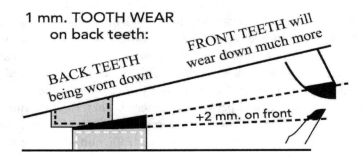

1 mm. TOOTH WEAR on back teeth:

FRONT TEETH will wear down much more

BACK TEETH being worn down

+2 mm. on front

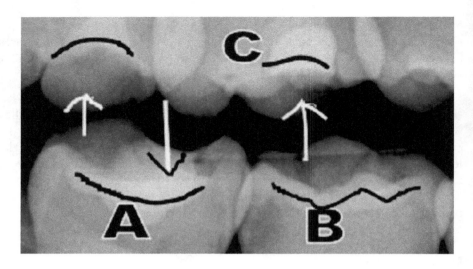

Fig. 3 Loss of Vertical

Tooth A: Has a large bowled-out filling caused by the upper cusp grinding against it, as shown by the middle row. Tooth B: Has a zig-zag line showing the shape of normal cups and has normal wear. It has a large cusp that's digging-out the white filling on Tooth C. On the left, Tooth A: Has a cusp grinding away the white filling at the at the end of the far-left arrow. This is what happens to white fillings that are too big. The mouth is collapsing due to the bowling-out of white fillings. These mild-to-severe cases can also happen to natural tooth structure or to gold when porcelain crowns are placed directly opposite them. In these cases, porcelain is so abrasive that it can grind away healthy teeth quickly.

THE HUMAN MOUTH & OCCLUSAL WEAR: The rate of wear often depends on the individual. The average woman for instance chews with less force and so will have less wear. Occlusal or Bite Collapse (Fig. 2 & 3) or loss of vertical height due to worn down fillings, crowns, and teeth is one of the most severe chronic problems of the mouth, as it requires extensive and expensive restorative work to correct. This is what we call "full mouth reconstruction." It will also tend to eventually break teeth and restorations and lead to open contacts and periodontal disease. Therefore, we must do all we can to offer the average patient a strong restoration which is reasonable in cost. Tough wear resistant restorations will save teeth, gums, and the mouth.

Dr. Hofmann often tells his patient not to replace metal fillings with weaker much more expensive tooth colored white fillings. The idea is to save the natural and shape and structure of your teeth and bite. Imagine the tip of your cusp hitting metal versus hitting the weaker white filling. The edge of the cusp will dig into the material. The large white filling will eventually bowl-out and lose its integrity as shown in the photo below. This allows the opposing cusp to dig deeper and deeper into the body of the filling. It can then break away the thinned-out walls of enamel.

If this digging-out happens on the main supporting teeth, you will lose the vertical length of both upper and lower teeth which is called "losing vertical." This also happens when a porcelain crown wears down the opposing weaker enamel. The x-ray on Figure 4, illustrates this type of collapse in a female patient who does not chew hard. It shows how much wear can happen in just a few years due to enamel cusps hitting the much weaker white filling. This wears down all the front teeth.

A good prevention against this type of wear is to place crowns of similar composition in direct opposition to each other, creating a "Stop or Stops" that will not wear down. If you plan to have multiple crowns done, you may want to ask your dentist about this. Gold should be placed against gold and porcelain against porcelain. This mechanical "stop" will help prevent wear on other teeth. In most cases, if the person has few crowns, it would be much better to leave the metal filling alone and seek to preserve as much of the natural tooth as a supportive surface. If the filling breaks, then replace it with a ceramic crown, inlay, *onlay*.

In America some dentists have moved away from placing amalgams because one of the ingredients in the mix is mercury. However, the American Dental Association declares amalgam is a safe filling material with some of the best margins in dentistry. If you have an old amalgam in your mouth, the weight of evidence shows mercury or mercury vapor is no longer present. The mercury was converted into an alloy when the dentist mixed it with silver, tin, copper, and zinc in a sealed container in his Amalgamator. The *amalgamation* process transforms the mercury into metal amalgam which in turn becomes super hard over a period of hours. The choice of what type of new restoration to use in your mouth will have more meaning to you as you continue to read on and understand chronic inflammation, the chewing forces of grinding, and the grave dangers of allowing periodontal disease to spread around the tooth. The restoration has to be strong and kind to the gums.

Dr. Hofmann states that he would rather have hundreds of old amalgams than one crown with open margins and inflamed gums like these below. One big problem is that decay will form undetected under the crowns (white) and bone loss will occur in the area, as shown in this x-ray of a perfect food trap for bacterial growth.

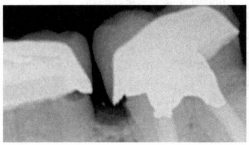

Figure 4.

The dentist who seeks perfection should design the crown with parallel walls for retention and tight margins in all areas. Unfortunately, just one area of open margin will collect food and irritate the gum tissue. Above is an excellent example of a what can go wrong with crowns: This set of two PORCELAIN TO METAL CROWNS IS A **PERFECT FOOD TRAP**. There is an open contact between the two molars, wide open margins under each crown, decay spreading through the left margin, and a huge hook-like overhang dooming the tooth on the right. As food slides between the teeth and under the overhang, the acids will build up and inter-dental bone will be destroyed. If decay spreads and reaches the nerve an abscess will form.

Evidence of problems is already apparent as shown by the above x-ray. Unless the crowns are removed and remade, decay will spread until the crowns fall off or a toothache occurs. By that time the bone will be further destroyed. Open contacts between molars allows for a great amount of damage to both bone and tooth. If you choose not to have expensive crowns, you will want strong fillings to preserve the vertical height of your teeth, and health of your gums. We will learn that weak fillings can allow vertical loss which will require the rebuilding of the bite. This is very expensive as it necessitates multiple crowns and bridges.

Chronic problems like periodontal disease and the enzymes they produce can become a great danger to the general health of a person. Research shows that those enzymes can damage the heart, pancreas and maybe vessels in the brain. These can threaten your life. Proper preventive techniques such as brushing, flossing, and mouth rinses will prevent and control the disease. Good saliva is key, and xylitol taken after meals and snacks is a great way to help it. Tight tooth contacts and the repair of decayed or broken teeth are extremely important to control bad bacteria. Effective mouth rinses for bone loss are the fluorides, chlorine dioxide, and chlorhexidine. Use them at night before you go to bed. Over-the-counter mouth rinses with essential oils, fluoride, or a zinc compound are very helpful for general use. Read Chapter 16, on how to use these tools to keep your mouth healthy.

Another serious problem related to the mouth and common to our pressurized society is Obstructive Sleep Apnea or OSA. As you sleep the airway collapses, blocking airflow. The person awakens over-and-over again gasping for air. In the process the body releases adrenaline which over time can raise the blood pressure. In time the heart weakens. Sleep apnea affects an estimated 22 million Americans and 80% of the moderate-to-severe cases will go undiagnosed. The American Sleep Apnea Association estimates that 38,000 in the U.S. alone die each year from heart disease directly related to sleep apnea.

The third life-threatening problem related to the mouth is the inhalation of bacteria infested plaque that collects around teeth in the elderly, weak, or bedridden patient. These patients are often unable to keep their molar teeth clean and can easily inhale the bacterial plaques around these teeth. Therefore, some dentists as a last resort advise removing the back molars. Another possible source for the pneumonia bacterium is from nasal drainage. Research is showing the xylitol can work against these and other bacterium, some of which can also cause periodontal disease. If you can stop periodontal disease, you may stop many of these life-threatening problems including dementia.

Another good idea is to provide caregivers a specially designed toothbrush with three interconnected brush heads to clean every surface at once. There are many brands available Online which can make brushing much easier for the caregiver. These also work for those who cannot use a regular toothbrush effectively.

You may also want to provide the nursing facility staff with a mouth rinse: one with essential oils that is anti-plaque or an activated chlorine dioxide rinse which can neutralize acids; or use both. Recommend a low carb-and-sugar diet and ask for a high fiber protein menu since it is too easy for senior facilities to serve empty carbs. If they serve candies, ask them to switch to non-sucrose candies such as xylitol mints which will protect their health. These come in many flavors. The brands with 240-250 mints in a jar are good. Plums, raspberries, mushrooms and strawberries also have xylitol. Have them start with small increments of xylitol and then work up to 15 grams.

Most of us and the elderly sweeten drinks with sugar or honey. Instead it is a great idea to provide xylitol packets to replace these cavity causing sugars. Xylitol protects the mouth from tooth decay and defeats bad microbes in both the gut and colon. It even prevents constipation while protecting the colon lining from cancer. It does this by neutralizing the yeast Candida Albicans and by lining the colon with n-butyrate which decreases leaks. What could be better?

The National Library of Medicine states that constipation or infrequent bowel movements is linked to an increased risk of cancer. The longer your waste or toxins are against the gut lining the more risk for carcinogenic activity. The recent scientific report, an analysis of 14 case–control studies, examined the relationship between constipation or infrequent bowel movements and colorectal cancer, uncovered a "statistically significant 48% increase in ratios for colorectal cancer in association with constipation." Wouldn't it be wise, therefore, to eat foods and food-medicines that will loosen the bowel movement while controlling bad bacteria or yeast in the mouth and the gut?

The Harvard Medical School study goes on to say, "If bad bacteria become dominant which can result when eating an unhealthy Western diet, or from exposure to pollution, medications and toxins then it can lead to an array of problems such as diarrhea, chronic constipation, irritable bowel syndrome and other serious diseases." Many doctors warn that these factors can also create a "leaky gut" syndrome which can then lead to many auto-immune diseases, weight gain, and other problems.

A simple way to prevent many of those problems is to preserve a healthy microbiome in both the gut and mouth. Inflammation in the gut is a result of an imbalance of bacteria just as it is in the mouth. This can be controlled by a good diet with prebiotics, probiotics and food medicines like xylitol. The research shows how interconnected the mouth is to the rest of the body. Therefore, the mouth is drawing more attention in the battle against pancreatitis, pancreatic cancer, pre-term births and infections of joints.

CHAPTER FOUR
<u>Challenges and Solutions</u>
Obsession with Bad habits

Has the pursuit of the perfectly, ultra-white, Hollywood smile enabled compulsive disorders and price-in-the-sky dentistry? Are we endangering the health of teeth by over whitening and over restoring? Parents who are trying to whiten their children's teeth should realize young teeth are much more vulnerable to sensitivity problems and to demineralization. Intense hydrogen peroxide can negatively affect the *cementum* attachment on roots which is important to preserve the delicate bone and tissue around the collar of each tooth.

The oral health of millions has been compromised by bad habits including illicit drugs, smoking, oral sex, chewing ice, and the use of tobacco products. Many cannot afford the Hollywood image and power treatments that are part of in-office whitening, implants, veneers, and crowns. Others cannot afford the consumption of empty calories in every form. A large portion of people cannot afford surgery and procedures to regenerate bone and tissue needed to correct defects, disease and recession. Even traditional procedures such as root canals, full dentures, and bridges are beyond the reach of many. Dental insurance, discount plans, or credit plans like Care Credit may be of some help.

Another option is to seek care at a Dental School or charity clinic. However, these choices are often limited or beyond the reach of many. These patients are often reluctant to see the dentist unless they are in pain or have another type of dental emergency. A fear of the dentist can block their desire to visit the dentist on a regular schedule. Some of these obstacles can be overcome with compassionate advice and information which this book offers.

The Pursuit of Profits

One comparison which will surprise many shows the average General Dentist makes more money than the General Physician. How can that be? Many nations pay physicians much more than dentists. Why the difference? My research points to cosmetic and implant dentistry. The cosmetic crown, veneer, and fillings, along with whitening, implants, and related devices are a huge market share of the dental business and will bring in huge profits. Unfortunately, the market overvalues these solutions and prices can be way out of the reach for many people. A simple cosmetic crown which costs the dentist an average lab cost of $130 or less to produce is delivered to the big city patient who has no insurance at an average charge of over $1000 with many charging over $1400. The high profit margin is a good reason for you to purchase a dental PPO insurance plan that covers crowns and can lower the cost to you by up to 70%.

Fears and Anxieties:

FEAR is an important factor keeping many people from going to the dentist and then following through with the treatment required. Fear can be initiated by memories from the past. If a dentist fails to pull back on the syringe when applying anesthetic, he or she may inject epinephrine into the blood stream which will then cause the patient's heart to rush or pump fast. Or if the needle hits a nerve it can cause an electrical jolt to the tongue. These experiences and others like this can initiate a fear of the dental chair!

If you have had pain during treatment, you may develop one of many symptoms including sweating, increased blood pressure and salivation, breathing difficulties, or choking.

This may set off a cascade of fear where symptoms occur one-after-another. If it turns into a panic attack, allergic reactions, syncope or fainting can occur. This scenario can haunt the patient and trigger future episodes when a needle is required. Therefore, every precaution should be taken to assure and comfort the fearful or distressed patient.

Women do seem to value dental visits and prevention more and may handle pain better. Many have a better understanding of dental procedures and their benefits. Some women have experienced the morning breath or bad breath of their partners. Having a better sense of smell, a woman will do more to keep her teeth clean of food and bacteria and will motivate their spouses to seek preventive care.

Dr. Hofmann likes to compare the fear phenomena to the aluminum foil test. A cook knows aluminum foil is not hot after it comes out of an oven. They know this from years of experience. The average person will think a heated piece of aluminum foil will burn their hands. The point is seeing a dentist is not as bad as your imagination dictates. Do not fear, for any pain you had as child was magnified by not only your lack of maturity, but also by the very fact the nerve centers in baby teeth and young permanent teeth are larger. As we grow older the nerve center of the tooth diminishes in size as calcium thickens the walls.

The adult tooth is unique in both its structure and its defense against infection. The tooth is not easily invaded by bacteria since it is protected by a very strong dentin-enamel matrix. If bacteria penetrate this barrier, which is as hard as topaz, the infection can destroy the living pulp tissue in the tooth, causing pain and requiring a root canal or extraction. A good diagram of a tooth and its bone socket is illustrated below. Refer back to this diagram as you read on. Figure 5

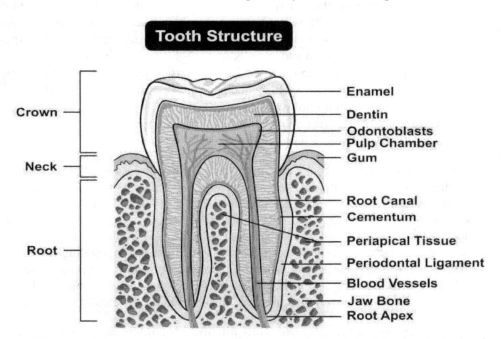

Nitrous Oxide may help some people overcome the initial fear and stress of going to the dentist. Nitrous is composed of one Oxygen atom and two Nitrogen atoms. Water is composed of one oxygen atom and two hydrogen atoms. This simple molecular structure makes nitrous oxide safe for the liver and the kidneys. The nitrogen atom is extruded through the skin in the same way sweat is. Nitrous acts as a muscle relaxant and therefore, can help anyone whose muscles tighten up when the mouth is be kept open too long. Nitrous may not be for everyone as it can make some people uncomfortable. Another help for those who have pain when leaving the mouth open for extended procedures is the mouth prop. Ask the dentist to place a small mouth prop in your mouth even for a tooth cleaning. This may also help any person that tends to dislocate their lower jaw. A child-size mouth prop is often the best solution. This will help the *temporal-mandibular joint* to relax. Study the diagram in Fig. 5 to help you understand your teeth.

False Thinking and Bad Information:

It is important to see the dentist on a regular basis for a checkup and cleaning, so you may gain important knowledge to prevent the dreaded toothache. If you do have pain, see the dentist as soon as possible! If you have tissue swelling, sensitivity usually increases, making it more difficult to numb the area. Swelling can also complicate the treatment and the healing. If your jaw swells, rinse often with warm water and salt and see a dentist as soon as possible. The heat helps to draw the infection out so it can drain while opening blood vessels to allow good blood cells in to fight the bad bacteria. The heat also draws the antibiotic into the area. Do NOT use a cold nor a hot compress outside the mouth, such as on the cheeks! This is part of the false thinking many people have. You do not want the infection to move outward into muscles and tissue. If you find surrounding muscle is hardening with infection, see your dentist quickly or go to an emergency room.

Just because you do not have pain, it doesn't mean you do not have a serious problem! Serious periodontal disease and other mouth infections often do not cause any pain, yet they can grow colonies of very bad bacteria producing enzymes that destroy bone and soft tissue. These enzymes can move into your blood stream and weaken your heart and other organs. Pain happens when a nerve is constricted, stretched, or under pressure. Bacteria penetrating the outer layer of a tooth can cause pain when it approaches or enters the pulp chamber called the pulp. Bacteria and its acids can cause the blood vessels and capillaries inside the chamber to swell thus pinching nerves. This is the classic toothache.

It is easy to be misinformed with all the false information flooding the marketplace. We place great trust in our friend's advice, media, education, perceptions, and what we learned growing up. Any or all of these could be wrong at any given time in our lives. And remember just because it is printed in your favorite magazine or proclaimed on television does not make it true nor good to use in your mouth or body. Big money and media hype do not guarantee that it will help you in the long term.

It may *Surprise You to Know* that a lifestyle combining a frequent use of apple cider vinegar, lemons, limes, or other forms of acid, can cause rampant decay in adults. In just one week, Dr. Hofmann had two patients with multiple areas of deep root decay caused by a daily apple cider vinegar regimen. Both claimed to be very hygiene conscious and yet both had extensive decay around the root and necks of many lower teeth. One was a new patient treating a respiratory issue and other had not been in for years thinking her recent apple cider habit would help her stomach. All they did was sip daily over many weeks or months apple cider vinegar to treat their problems. Constant sipping will dilute and acidify your precious saliva. Our goal is to cultivate good non-acidic saliva and healthy bacteria for a self-cleaning attractive mouth.

There are over 500 drugs and over-the-counter medications that decrease salivary flow. This dryness can cause major problems for both the oral cavity and the sinuses. Xylitol, however, can decrease this dryness while controlling bad bacteria in the mouth and in nasopharyngeal areas? Many nurses in hospitals know how effective xylitol is in breaking down congestion and healing sinusitis. Yet few of us have been informed. Why is this? Is it because big pharma or retail business interests feel it will hurt their business? Halitosis, constipation, middle ear infections and many other problems are helped or cured with xylitol. Chlorine dioxide also neutralizes acidic saliva, halitosis, and many of conditions already mentioned. Plus it can kill spores and bad bacteria.

Solution #1: XYLITOL "The Wonder Molecule":

One shortcoming in America is we rarely do bottom-up evidence generated research. Media coverage on preventive medicine or products such as xylitol and activated chlorine dioxide is non-existent. One reason may be because research is very expensive and there is little corporate backing for anything that does not benefit them. The American Dental Association (ADA) for instance says it cannot afford the cost of independent research without some corporate backing. Xylitol, clove oil and activated chlorine dioxide are not profit makers for dental and medical retail corporations. They typically will not sponsor research in these areas. Thus, most research done on the effectiveness of xylitol in combating tooth decay, sinus and ear infections is being done in other countries where they do listen to personal testimonies of healing from food-medicines. Research in Japan and China is showing that xylitol can heal serious problems such as cancer and flu. Research in Canada indicates it improves bone density in animals.

Studies in Finland spanning many decades show that giving children xylitol gum three times per day, after each meal and after school, can eliminate the formation of tooth decay in children. This 61-year study with thousands of children and adults is one of the most extensive scientific studies ever done in the world. And it began as a dental study. The Finnish government kept careful records revealing that xylitol from birch trees made a big difference in the health of the population. This research was totally unbiased since it was NOT paid for by special interests nor corporations. This should draw your attention!

One study of high-risk pregnant women found a profound decrease of decayed teeth in both mothers and their newborn children up to the age of five. The mothers chewed xylitol gum 3 times per day before and after their pregnancy. The scientists discovered there was a decrease in transmission from mother to child of a key bacterium causing tooth decay. In these studies, Finnish scientists discovered there was also a 42% decrease in ear infections. Again, these studies involve a large sampling of people over decades since World War II. Have you heard about these discoveries? This wonder molecule protected children as young as five from tooth decay, nasal congestion and middle ear infections.

These studies were of interest to Dr. A. H. "Lon" Jones MD, a rural doctor who tried xylitol on his kids and patients both as a preventive and as a solution to treat sinusitis and many other ailments. Unlike the Finnish study, he used it as an external spray application, and It worked so well even adults with chronic rhinosinusitis and kids with middle ear infections were effectively healed. We now know its effectiveness in decreasing weight gain, intra-ocular pressures in the eye, and the severity of chronic wounds. It may also help prevent glaucoma.

Apparently, there is no real downside to its use. If you consume too much it will pass through your system acting as a prebiotic and protection for your colon against cancer. Too much, however, can produce runny stools. One research paper stated that taking 130 grams in a day would cause diarrhea. It is safe for diabetics but talk to your doctor and start with a small amount such as one or two grams three times per day. It is available in granular form or as a mint or gum.

Studies show chewing gum with a mix of sorbitol and xylitol also reduces acidity of the saliva and therefore can control the bad bacteria. A gentle spray of xylitol can maintain the health and native immunity of both nasal and oral mucosa. Unlike nasal flushes which have become so popular, this solution does not remove the good mucosal layer. Nasal flushes using plain water can dry out nasal passages allowing dust particles and bacteria to create a *mucositis infection*. Therefore, some people are adding xylitol to their nasal rinses for added protection.

Xylitol can help those who have dryness issues in the mouth caused by mouth breathing or the over-use of certain medicines. Xylitol stimulates the production of saliva and the thinning out of congestion in the nasal passages. This dilutes toxins and acids, then washes away the bad bacteria. It also stops that bad bacteria from damaging tissue and protects the good bacteria around teeth, gums, and sinuses. This is much better than depending on antibiotics. Because xylitol is non-fermentable, bacteria cannot be converted into acid. Instead xylitol helps to provide a safe non-acidic saliva and nasal phlegm. For those with persistent oral dryness there are new products such as "XyliMelts" which dispenses xylitol slowly to moisturize the mouth. Since xylitol is semi-absorbable it will eventually work its way into the gut where it stimulates fluid flow defeating constipation.

Physiologically xylitol works against bacteria in two powerful ways. 1. As the bad bacteria consumes the 5-carbon sugar they cannot metabolize the sugar into acids. 2. The inactivated bacteria are then compelled to detach from mucosal and tooth surfaces preventing them from attacking tissue cells directly. They are no longer protected by their attachment to decalcified teeth or to swollen tissue.

Amazingly, xylitol also stimulates the flow of saliva which helps wash away the bacteria. These opportunistic bacteria such as Strep mutants are effectively removed without hurting the good bacteria. The saliva can now return to a healthy pH level. Compare this to weed control lawn fertilizer and its ability to protect "good grass" while disabling bad fast-growing weeds. The good grass is left alone much like good cells, bacteria, and fibroblasts are preserved by xylitol. Unfortunately, smoking and other stimulants such as vaping can harm many of those good cells and increase acidity of the saliva which will help the bad bacteria multiply in numbers.

Another amazing attribute of xylitol is that up to 15 grams is being produced daily in the mitochondria of our cells. Why is it stored in this key part of every cell? Both mitochondrial RNA and DNA, incorporate the 5-carbon sugar ribose in their long chain. They help identify who you are and act as the factory for repair and building cells and tissue. What does the 5-carbon xylitol do in this metabolic process? Xylitol does have the ability to carry calcium ions wherever needed. Research indicates that this unique multipurpose molecule may play an integral role in cellular metabolism for both plant and animal kingdoms.

As a 5-Carbon sugar xylitol appears to flow freely throughout the body passing through the gut, placenta and bone barriers while causing no harm. So, why is it taking so long for both physicians and dentists to recognize this amazing molecule? Although researched worldwide and used by nurses in hospitals, few doctors here realize how effective xylitol is as a preventative and cure for diseases like Strep throat. It acts as a medicine unlike artificial sweeteners which may have long term harmful effects. So why do most large grocers carry every kind of sugar and sugar substitute except for xylitol?

Research shows that the long-term effects of xylitol is good. We know that it stops constipation, and if stools get too loose, just cut back on the dose. This can happen to people who eat too much too quickly or have an allergic reaction to sugar alcohols, which is rare. Be cautious if you have had part of your colon removed or have chronic diarrhea for any reason. Xylitol is a carbohydrate with 40% less calories than regular sugar and it has a very low glycemic index. When replacing regular sugar, it can help the diabetic maintain stable blood sugar and insulin levels.

We now have an ample supply of xylitol since it is being extracted from discarded corn cobs. We are fortunate to have a safe and cheap resource for xylitol. Corn cobs are an abundant natural waste product. Is it possible that corn cobs were used as toothbrushes by American Indians and other early civilizations? Were there other easy sources of xylitol in foods? Was it a natural food-medicine?

One unnatural sugar substitute recommended for diabetics is sucralose (Splenda) which is a non-nutritive sweetener, meaning it provides no dietary calories. It is considered a high-intensity sugar which is hundreds of times sweeter than sugar. However, sucralose is made by replacing three natural carbon to hydrogen and oxygen bonds with three chlorine atomic bonds. This molecule is now a chlorocarbon as is DDT, and therefore, is of concern to scientists. Fructose sugar which is often promoted by juicing is also problematic, since it is metabolized in the liver, where the excess fructose is converted into fat or triglycerides.

On the next page is a chart that will summarize the extraordinary multi-functional role that xylitol plays in physiology and health. It shows that xylitol helps to prevent colon cancer in two ways: It controls the yeast Candida Albicans and it converts excess xylitol into butyrate which then protects the colon. Xylitol also helps protect the mouth in 4 different ways: 1) Inactivates bad bacteria, 2) Detaches the bad bacteria from teeth and inflamed surfaces, 3) Stimulates saliva flow which will dilute the acids, and 4) Helps to heal demineralized enamel. It's a perfectly symmetrical molecule that can also carry calcium to strengthen bone.

Used as a preventative, xylitol can save lives. A prime bad bacterium that causes serious gum inflammation and destruction in the mouth is *Porphyromonas gingivalis*, or *P. gingivalis*. It can be found in joints, heart plaques, and in the placenta. Scientists believe it is carried there through the blood stream from the mouth and therefore, prior to a cleaning people with joint replacements should take antibiotics. Controlling this bacteria in the mouth will foster a healthy saliva and can save lives including that of the fetus.

Multi-Functional XYLITOL	Activity or Purpose	Other Special Benefits
Xylitol is produced and stored in the Mitochondria, the cells factory...	For the purpose of calcium transport or for the repair or defense of the cell.	It's Tridentate ligand, [H-C-OH]$_3$ allows it to carry calcium ions across the cell wall.
Xylitol consumed by pregnant mothers....	"Inoculates" fetus and baby protecting up to the age of 5 from tooth decay.	Helps to protect the bacterial flora of the mother and the fetus.
Xylitol consumed as a mint, gum or raw like sugar by children as young as 5 or by adults and the elderly.	Protects mouth-throat-nasal mucosa, gut lining, and teeth from bad bacteria. Keeps microbiome healthy & prevents tooth decay.	Decreases acidity of saliva & intraocular pressures that cause glaucoma. Helps heal decalcifications on teeth and bone.
Xylitol dissolved in water or in a saline solution and used as a mouth spray....	Works directly on Strep mutans, other bad bacteria, and Candida to prevent or intercept infections.	Labeled sugar-free by retailers it has a low glycemic index of 7 versus 70 for sucrose.
Xylitol dissolved in saline with essential oils for nasal squirt....	Liquifies heavy nasal congestion and stops bad bacteria.	Helps break up heavy salt mucus in airway lining of cystic fibrosis patients.
Xylitol eaten in fruit and vegetables....	Digested by intestines helps probiotics work, as it stops bad bacteria	Also contributes fiber which helps GI tract and microbiome.
Excess xylitol is converted to butyrate in colon which the liver can convert to ketose..	Lines the colon wall protecting it from Candida Albicans and colon cancer. Has slight allergy potential. Start slow and is safe for us but not dogs.	Stops constipation but, if you take too much too quickly it can cause a runny stool. Start with 5 to 10 grams which is 2 tsps. and go to 15.

Why has the general public not heard about the benefits of chewing xylitol gum and mints, or spraying the nose with a xylitol mist? Although accepted in Europe, corporate America does not use nor promote xylitol and therefore does little research on it. Many large grocers do not carry xylitol gum, mints nor powder, yet they devote a wide space to Stevia, Splenda, Equal and Sweet-n-low. Research on xylitol's amazing benefits spans 61 years among 100's of thousands of people in all age groups throughout the world; but little of this research is done in America.

In preparing for this book very few doctors who conversed with Dr. Hofmann knew anything about the power of xylitol. However, nurses he spoke to said they used it in the hospital. This may be explained by the fact the nurses are more involved in the day to day care of patients whereas physicians acting as overseers may be too distracted to notice the healing power of xylitol.

Dr. Hofmann is not surprised by this failure since he made the mistake years ago in buying some xylitol spray which he then left unused and unsold in his cabinet. The logic of using sugar to heal problems caused by sugar does not register easily in one's mind. He now calls xylitol a "wonder molecule" and now uses it on a regular basis as a mint, chewing gum, and to sweeten coffee. Amazingly, it stimulates the flow of fluids: saliva in the mouth, the dilution of phlegm or mucus in the nasal passages, and the softening of stools in the colon. Research shows that it decreases the concentration of salts in the airway surface fluids which affect people suffering from cystic fibrosis.

In conclusion this amazing substance works internally as a preventive and externally as a healing agent hindering both bad bacteria and the cancer producing yeast *Candida Albicans*. Regular 6-carbon sugar stimulates the growth of both the bad bacteria and bad yeast whereas the 5-carbon Xylitol works to stop them. Xylitol protected the Finnish children against potential ear, nose, and throat problems. The initial study began 81 years ago and now involves a population of people from birth to death. We have learned that xylitol is so unique companies label it a "sugar free" sugar which makes no sense, yet our FDA seems to agree.

Dr. Hofmann found that a spray of xylitol directed at the tissue can work better and quicker than his penicillin pills to heal severe inflammation in the throat.

Solution # 2: Silver Diamine Fluoride is another treatment that has had great success overseas. SDF has been effectively used in countries like Australia for over 5 years to defeat decay in children, but we only recently started research here to allow for its approval by the FDA. Many third world countries have been using it on their children for over three years. Yet few people here know about this decay destroying chemical that works without the use of a needle or drill.

Solution # 3: Preventive Education and Care concepts in other countries are very effective. Brazilian dentistry was greatly influenced by pioneer American dentists who migrated to Brazil after the Civil War. Their dental care begins at an early age in schools where problems are caught early, and prevention is emphasized. The dentist-to-total population ratio is one the best in the world. We can also learn from dentistry performed in Europe, Australia, and Asia. In Europe or the EU there is an official recognition of the preventive medical and dental value of xylitol. They also emphasize the use of oral appliances to expand the jaw or palate in order to make room for erupting permanent teeth. They understand that expansion creates a bigger airspace for breathing and a broader more attractive smile line.

American dentistry has traditionally pushed the idea of extracting two or four Bicuspids in a narrow arch. In the past this did not seem important, but now we know how important it is to enlarge the airspace in the mouth for good non-obstructed breathing. Shrinking the mouth by extracting teeth in a growing teenager's mouth may shape a beautiful small arch, but it may also increase the potential for sleep disorders. At this point more studies need to be done.

Dr. Hofmann loves the profession of dentistry and believes many dentists have become so merchandise and profit oriented that median prices for many dental procedures are way too high. Prevention has taken a back seat instead of being part of the treatment. Dentists should be warning you about hidden sugars that cause tooth decay. For instance, one teaspoon of ketchup has 4 grams of sugar! Yogurt with fruit is full of sugar and one average slice of chocolate cake can have as many as 24 teaspoons. High concentrations of fructose from both juicing and HFCS can lead to a fatty liver. All this points to the fact that one in three adults in America rank as being pre-diabetic.

If you feel your dental visit is like the "in-and-out" fast-food experience, let the dental office know. During your last visit did you learn anything about your unique mouth that will help you prevent problems or disease? Did you have a meaningful discussion with the staff - one that gave you a "I did not know that" moment? Did they just try to sell you stuff or were you able to ask the right questions?

CHAPTER FIVE
Challenges of the Modern
Dentist

Modern dentistry has changed to such a degree it may seem to be more like an engineering science than a medical science. This trend has made the dental office much more expensive to furnish and design. In turn the cost of treatment for patients has increased and continues to rise. When Dr. Hofmann started his dental practice, he had very little debt, and invested about $65,000 to buy and equip his practice. However, today's high-tech dental office often includes the very expensive electronic equipment with prices shown below:

Cancer detection devices: $1000-6,500. Electronic Bite Registration + CAD CAM: $3000-84,500

Digital Impression Scanner $9,900-19,900.   Digital X-ray for one operatory is over $35,000

Digital Extra-oral Imaging: $42,000- 240,000.   Milling machines for crowns: $25,000- 90,000.

Note these costs do not include the overall costs of staffing, design and installation, energy & water, general lighting & phone systems, air compressor-dryers, bathroom and reception areas, and the signage along with special interior decorations and branding.

There are many other specialized devices including: root apex detectors, high range curling lights, Electronic Periodontal Probes, intra-oral cameras, communication systems, computers with their backup systems, shade detectors, panoramic x-rays = $15,000 to $50,000. This does not include the cost for the basic equipment: surgical lights, dental chairs, dental cabinets, nitrous oxide with oxygen plumbing = $35,000 to $75,000 to each operator. Add another $8,000 to $30,000 for bleaching or Whitening lights, inventory for hundreds of treatment procedures, lab equipment, utility equipment such as suction and compressor systems, and office supplies to run an effective dental practice; along with advertising. The above does not include the daily expenses which add up quickly if a dentist is trying to start up a practice. Today's dental office can easily cost 2-4 times what Dr. Hofmann paid.

A recent report suggests young dentists have on average a 75% overhead. This means three out of four dollars that he or she makes goes to paying debts and the overhead of running the practice.

The ADEA (American Dental Education Association) says the average debt per dental school graduate is $287,331 (according to a 2017 survey). The original idea of educating a wide variety of students was to motivate many of them to practice in many of the small towns throughout America. It is easy to understand why many of these students cannot afford to do this in today's financial climate. Therefore, new dentists should either associate with another dentist or start out small, equipping their office with basic needs.

Of all the professions, the modern dental office is by far the most difficult and expensive to plumb and equip. This may be the reason why most dentists do not move into rural areas where dentists are most needed. Many feel they can make more profit in the big city. Frankly, money more than ever seems to be driving dentistry. Many graduates are joining large groups or a Dental Services Organization (DSO). The Sept. 2018, publication of the "Dental Products Report" states 60% of dentists are part of a group practice or DSO. Of those surveyed over 70% believe the trend will increase. Yet when rating their jobs from a scale of 1 to 10 those who rated it 6 or below were the majority!

The biggest complaint was the lack of continuity of care where one doctor was not able to start and finish a treatment for a given patient. This could also be tough on the patient who does not know who will be treating them on their next visit and whether the new dentist understands their special needs and will follow through with what the other dentist said. The same study showed 73% of potential graduates from dental school want to join a group or dental services organization and not create their own practice. This seems to be the trend for the future and could drive out the small family practice. Unfortunately, this also forebodes higher prices to continue as competition is diminished.

The increase in population and the advancement of technology are also driving dentistry towards unchartered horizons. What are the answers? One suggestion is for new dentists to trim their overhead so they can have a buffer zone for success. Another is to increase the new dentists from here and abroad until prices for everything comes down. So far, neither idea has lowered prices.

Now a suggestion being made by the government and medical community is for every dental office to have sophisticated software to communicate with both hospitals and physicians. Although expensive for the small practice this concept would help create a seamless strategy to handle chronic diseases of the mouth between both the medical and dental communities. It would enable physicians to more effectively predict and treat heart disease and other disorders diagnosed in dental offices.

These technological demands and the expansion of Dental Service Organizations may end up being the wave of the future which controls prices in the health community, but swamps the small private practice driving them out of business. It will tie the dentist and patient to the physician and related hospital tests. And it will favor the large corporate or group practices that have huge budgets and can afford these upgrades. It will hurt the small solo-practice and again, this will eventually increase the cost of dental care for everyone and may end the traditional private practice.

A big concern is that these added pressures and the lack of effective controls may lead to more market oriented dentistry with less attention to ethics and service. It seems that in almost every arena in this modern era we have more lies and deception. Popular thinking generates myths and misconceptions that foment fear and bad thinking. Two good examples are the fluoride and mercury fears both of which can generate big profits for those who merchandise products and services that cater to them. They bring up Nazi research that supposedly created explosive fluorine (which has very little to do with the fluoride in water) and a theory that Hitler used fluoride to dumb down the Jews. This is a complete myth. Chlorine gas is deadly, yet we put extra chlorine in swimming pools and we still swim in them? Chlorine is not removed with water filters, yet we continue to drink both city and bottled water. The mercury fear has been used to attack the super-hard Amalgam alloy, yet we consume large amounts of tuna and feed it to kids. Don't let fear drive your thinking. This kind of hyper-information may not affect you, but it can others.

In determining what is true and what is not we should use a good "Truth Filter." One should evaluate the preponderance of evidence by non-biased, double-blind studies and not just accept the conclusions of a talking-head on a video. The products used by Root-canal specialists in doing root canals, for instance, are inert and safe - they cannot poison you. This book is based on good research not paid for by corporate interests. Dr. Hofmann has not received any financial benefit from any company. He is not receiving any money for any product, but does recommend those that can help you.

CHAPTER SIX
<u>Naked or High-Tech</u>
Super-Dentist

When Dr. Hofmann started his dental career, he felt that if he did not keep up with the latest technology, he would be left naked and behind. So, after a few years, he bought the latest High-Tech dental equipment, and most were wise decisions. However, there was one space-age tool that was expensive and almost useless. This was the dental laser which proved to be intimidating to both patients and assistants alike. It did very little to improve the care of the patient! Now there are ten times as many types of super-expensive devices.

One solution is for dental labs to operate these costly machines and therefore spread the cost of operation among dentists who use them. Why fill up dental offices with multiple complicated pieces of equipment which require dedicated trained staff members to run them and maintain them? Why would a dentist want to buy complicated machinery to then feel helpless when it malfunctions, or when a special part or shade selection is no longer in the inventory? Why not let the large dental labs make the big investments and share their expensive and intensive inventory with their client dentists? They can economically buy in lots and train people to run the machines day in and day out? They have the ability to generate very cosmetic and accurate crowns.

The truth is the manufacturers and corporate supply companies do NOT want this. They want to make the profitable sale and will try everything to motivate that young dentist to spend and invest in their expensive equipment. These are some of the same complex challenges the medical community has faced for many years. The costly devices and drugs add a lot to the dramatic increase in the price of healthcare. Expensive tests are pushing the envelope of insurance coverage. When is another test, x-ray or special ionizing scan not necessary?

In dentistry a classic toothache without a *peri-apical abscess* can create challenges. Normally if you had on-and-off pain a digital x-ray is taken, and hot or cold tests are done to see if the tooth is dead or dying from an internal injuries or infection. If the tests and x-ray did not clearly indicate the need for a root canal, the bite is checked, and adjusted if needed. In today's world, however, the patient may find their dentist referring them to the *Endodontist* for *an expensive ionizing scan* called a 3-D Cone-Beam ionizing scan.

Today's Endodontist has many great tools to save what may have been called a hopeless tooth a few years ago. Regenerative techniques can save many of those badly abscessed or loose teeth. However, in some instances, dental insurance companies will demand an extraction. They can block a treatment that does not fit their protocol. They could demand an implant and reject the dentist's treatment plan which calls for a root canal and crown. The implant specialist may then need another ionizing scan called the CBCT scan to map out the bone for implant placement. This means more radiation on the head.

An even more difficult diagnosis is detecting a crack. A regular x-ray usually can only detect the cracks which have spread beyond the root and into the bone. The 3-D Cone Beam scan can detect a crack in the tooth that has not penetrated the bone nor the pulp. The best treatment for dangerous cracks is often a temporary or stainless-steel crown. It may prevent the crack from advancing. Later a permanent crown can be done. Hopefully your dental insurance will see it that way and accept this provisional treatment plan.

The best High-Tech investment Dr. Hofmann made was buying a digital x-ray unit. He was one of the first dentists in his metro area to acquire the Schick Digital X-ray System which was the original digital dental x-ray developed by the U.S. Navy for ship to shore transmission. Prior to digital we had to wait ten to fifteen minutes for development of the x-ray and then we were lucky if it turned out perfect. Often the analog x-rays were too light or too dark due to stale chemicals, bad temperatures, or equipment malfunction. Digital x-rays are instantaneous, accurate, easily transmitted over distance, and produces much less energy with 6 times less radiation exposure to the patient. It allows the dentist to quickly confirm the fit of crowns, bridges, and the length of roots for proper root canal sealing. And if you need a copy of the x-ray to take with you for a second opinion, it should be free, since paper copies are easy to make!

Dr. Hofmann has enjoyed being both a professional artist and dentist. As a service to his patients he does not believe in charging a premium price. He has kept his fees at or below median levels for his area. Dr. Hofmann prefers "personality" in a Smile and NOT "white-perfection." He has seen many "chicklet smiles" that are obviously fake and draw the eyes to the teeth and not the overall beauty of the face and the natural smile. He shares this because he has seen many poorly fitting crowns that are unattractive. Promoting super-white teeth is not healthy to teeth, just as promoting super-slim bodies is not healthy to the body. And as an artist and dentist he prefers natural beauty.

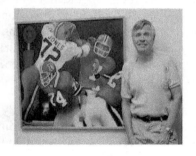

The artist-dentist posing by his photo-realistic painting of Superbowl XII painted in acrylic on canvas.

As stated earlier, he graduated from the University of Texas Health Science Center in San Antonio which had the fortune of drawing many of the top dental professionals from a talented pool of military officers in the Armed Services. Many of them were authors of the technical books used in teaching dentistry throughout the country. They taught a very conservative way of saving and restoring teeth. One of those techniques is the 3-step procedure to remove tooth decay ending with a delicate hand instrument called a spoon excavator to remove the final layers of decay. This decreases the chance of overheating the core nerve in the tooth and helps to prevent accidental nerve exposure with drills. It also ensures the last bit of decay will be removed!

Another conservative concept is using Silver Diamine Fluoride to remove decay without having to use a needle or drill. With SDF a dentist can drill at an angle between teeth and not have to weaken the vulnerable support on top. This conservative approach will save the strength of the tooth and the patient both time and money. It will do away with those weak tooth-colored fillings.

The dental graduate has big bills to pay and therefore must learn to manage money and budgets before they get out of control. They need to start small with less debt and better cost control. They should not allow themselves to be tempted by all the gadgets the dental industry wants to sell them. It is easy to rack up tens of thousands of dollars in debt and then spend tens of thousands more to try to attract new patients.

Each year these costs increase & the challenge of attracting new patients becomes more competitive and difficult.

Dentistry and those charged with taking care of patients should be held more accountable to standards of education where the patients understanding is more important than selling of treatments and products. The focus should not be on production goals, the bonus plans, motivational huddles, the selling of cosmetic concepts, and the latest creative profit-making sales pitches. Dr. Hofmann advises people who have doubts about any product or treatment, not to buy it, but to wait and if necessary, get a second opinion or check it out online. Go to Pub Med or Medline or other online sites for ideas and good research.

Information on unethical practices in dentistry is rarely discussed openly either as a professional courtesy or as an unspecified covenant within the professional community. Some doctors may feel it will hurt the image of dentistry. Do you believe habitual scamming should be exposed so that the public can evaluate and judge all facts and circumstances? Where are the reporters? Are they afraid of losing advertising profits or of being sued?

Can the public help motivate the profession of dentistry to change for the better? For instance, we have an aging population that will need a lot of special care. Despite all the warnings and the incorporation of specially trained staff, thousands upon thousands of elderly in nursing facilities die each year due to unclean teeth and bacteria plaques being inhaled. The teeth are not being cleaned by the staff nor by these incapacitated patients. The dental plaque carries colonies of gram-negative bacteria that can cause deadly pneumonia. And this is the number one cause of death in these facilities. Can a good diet plus xylitol help remedy this dire situation? Who will step up?

Being a doctor is a privilege and every dentist should stand by the Hippocratic Oath with both a promise to do the patient no harm and a desire to heal and not seek gain from a patient's vulnerability or lack of knowledge. The patient must have faith in our health system. Therefore, the focus should be on truthful and honest teaching, treating, guiding and reporting.

Healthcare needs to refocus its effort to incorporate all means of effective and safe preventive medicine. Instead of focusing on profits and cost we should focus on what has worked best in various countries. Dr. Hofmann states, "during my recent attendance at a renowned international presentation the biggest study focused on just one country, the country from which a major corporation gave substantial financial support. These studies do not help us determine the best solutions. They are too narrow focused and biased. We need to do comparative studies on the successes coming from many countries around the world. By working together, we can beat ever-increasing rates of auto-immune and bacteria-led diseases. Forget the profits and frivolous marketing.

CHAPTER SEVEN
Understanding the Problem

According to many parameters, dentistry is one of the best professions to step into. The entrance exams are some of the easiest, the average income is high, and the work hours when dictated by the self-employed dentist, range from a 3-day to 5-day week, and rarely require more than 35 hours per week. In the 2019 ranking of the 100 Best Jobs, *U.S. News and World Report* gave the career "Dentist" the fourth highest spot and the #2 spot for best health care job.

The stress level in modern dentistry is minimal and the hazards have been greatly reduced. The average American Family Physician, however, makes less money than the average American Family Dentist. Is this fair considering the risks, the hours worked, the extra years of internship, and general complexity of knowledge required to diagnose and treat the whole body compared to just the mouth? The cost of malpractice insurance for a physician can vary from three to over 6 times higher than the general dentist! Compared to a registered nurse, the dental hygienist also has amazing advantages. Some of the challenges for a Registered Nurse are as follows:

1) They must go through intensive training in and out of hospitals.
2) She or he has far more responsibilities and risks.
3) With that comes more stress and more demands in adapting to changes in medicine. Their continuing education is much more intensive.
4) They work grave yard hours and must deal with hospital protocol, hospital administrative policies, and a wide variety of doctors and staff members with their demanding egos and personalities.
5) The RN must know more, do more, and lift more weight to help and care for bedridden patients. They face more life and death situations with a much more risk to their own health and well being. Some must be prepared for tough cases like burn victims and a variety of unknown diseases and challenges.

The average gross salary of a hygienist was $68,440 in 2016 according to *U.S. News & World Report*. It may not include the bonuses they make for selling various treatments and products such as "Tooth Whitening," "Ultra-Sonic toothbrushes", and other non-essential cosmetic items. That same year *U.S. News & World Report* stated in a BLS report (Bureau of Labor Statistics showing the RN average pay was $68,450/year. The hygienist works less than 33 hours per week. The July 15, 2018, *Payscale Report* says the average hourly wage for neonatal nurses was $29.31 per hour vs the hygienist $33.33 per hour. And like physicians an RN has a higher malpractice cost.

The hygienist is a professional and deserves a good salary. With this, however, must come a professional dedication to teaching and serving the patient. All the selling and marketing of ultra-sonic toothbrushes, power flossers, cosmetic solutions, and other devices may distract the patient from what they need to learn and do in order to prevent and control periodontal disease in an effective way. It may also distract the professional from doing a thorough exam with the necessary instructions and guidelines.

The bonus system can be a big benefit for the hygienist. Unfortunately, the bonus incentive is often used to motivate both hygienist and dentists to work faster, see more patients, sell more treatments, and promote more products. These Madison avenue concepts can also lead to the promotion of unnecessary services and inflated prices. This book will help guide you during your next visit. Are you attracted to T.V ads promoting "Sexy Teeth?" Do you think these market driven systems are good for you and for dentistry?

Learning is key. There are simple techniques that can greatly benefit you. Using two toothbrushes will work to keep each dry and prevent re-contamination by bacteria? Drying the bristles thoroughly or using soap will kill the bacteria. A germ-controlled environment will cultivate a healthy saliva. This is a recommendation Dr. Ellie Phillips makes in her new book, *Mouth Care Comes Clean*. She states, "Mouth health is determined by a delicate balance that is under our control each day, for better or worse." In her book she suggests our preventive protocols may be misplaced, and we should focus on preserving a healthy oral biofilm with a saliva that encourages tooth recalcification and healing. Chapter twenty-three will cover this more.

If you have tooth enamel erosion or rotated teeth and other food traps try using a Korean type super-soft toothbrush in those areas, and a second regular soft brush for the other areas. Never use a medium or hard brush. Mechanical toothbrush manufacturers often claim their products churn up or vibrate saliva and therefore clean better. They show this in television ads. The mouth is not a swimming pool and "NO," they do not churn up saliva. They can do harm since their bristles are often stiffer than a good soft or super-soft bristle. A hand-held super-soft bristle bends with the curve of both the tooth and bone allowing bristles to bend around and massage the fragile tissue at the neck or collar of teeth. The bristles can then penetrate food traps without harming healthy tissues.

Have you seen the spinning circular brush-head of a street-sweeper? Now imagine it sweeping against a white picket fence. It will strip the wood and paint. The spinning toothbrush bristles hit the thin collar tissues like a street-sweepers bristles hitting a white fence. The angle of contact is destructive. Hopefully your hygienist will take the time to show you how to gently wipe the collar and side of teeth with a back and forth action. The ADA provides standard diagrams on how to brush at a 45-degree angle to the collar of the gum tissue.

As we dig deeper and expose more "naked truths" you will appreciate the need to understand Preventive Medicine. Many of us have been exposed to ideas and concepts tailored by American companies and their research studies. We know little about products like xylitol which were discovered and researched in other countries. Even though xylitol has saved the health of millions at a very low cost per capita, the American public knows very little about it. And what the public is told is subtly negative. We are warned that it can harm dogs or cause diarrhea (which it rarely does.) Yet facts show it is widely used in Finland without negative effects on an entire population of kids. Instead we choose to depend on a list of big pharma drugs that can have many severe bad effects. And the same is true for the synthetic sugars. We take these substances by faith, hoping they will not cause harm to our organs and tissues.

Why do major grocery chains still carry a wide variety of sugar and sugar substitutes except for xylitol? Is this a bias due to lack of demand? Or are the sugar cartels suppressing it? Xylitol's power has been known for decades! Big money would lose huge profits in many markets including laxatives and the ear-nose-and-throat market. Our health system spends more money than any nation in the world on sugar, alcohol and drugs. Drug companies waste billions of dollars on marketing, and lobbying and buying Congressional leaders. The point is prevention and food-medicines do not line pockets and are not big money makers. Will we choose to be dependent on disease for economic prosperity? Is it too late to break this perpetual cycle of disease and waste?

Many European dental societies endorse the use of xylitol and promote it for public health. Instead of selling expensive devices, Botox treatments, sexy teeth or spa concepts outside of dentistry, dental offices should be teaching and promoting good preventive measures and concepts to stop disease. Dr. Hofmann hears a lot of complaints from people he interviews concerning the forced merchandising of products. Patients have to deal with a barrage of sales pitches.

Our dental and medical industry needs to learn from two small town doctors who created the world's greatest medical institution that is now a worldwide institution of hope and science. The Mayo Clinic motto is *"Faith, Hope, and Science."* Each doctor is paid a salary that is not based on the number of surgeries or the number of patients seen.

There is NO monetary motivation for them to complete treatments quickly, to see more patients, nor to sell more tests. They devote their time and energy to serving and treating each patient with diligence. Like the spokes of a wheel each field of medicine is focused on the patient who is in the center.

The Mayo brothers developed the heart-lung bypass machine and were the first to position pathology labs in proximity to operating rooms. Mayo includes over 4,700 staff physicians and research scientists treating 1.3 million patients from all 50 states and 136 countries. They do not receive any royalties for the inventions, technology, or concepts developed. Not too long ago, Dr. Hofmann had the opportunity to join an important medical mission with some Mayo Clinic surgeons and their staff. A group of these selfless men and women paid their own way to provide free care for widows and orphans in the high mountains of what is called the IXIL Triangle in northern Guatemala. By God's grace he was part of this miracle mission which will be discussed in more detail later as we explore answers to good oral health.

CHAPTER EIGHT
The Driven vs. the Guided
Protecting Your Health

Driven people versus guided people: this does not preclude being a little of both. On Dr. Hofmann's way home, he looked to his right as a fancy black sports car with dark tinted windows jerked onto the right lane which had a white curved arrow warning of lane-merging. Certainly, this person should have seen the car ahead of his was going slow, but the determined individual decided to gain 20 ft. by darting ahead and grabbing the small gap ahead. All done for what? The driven personality often does not care, all he or she wants to do is get ahead. We see the wrecks of driven people and their victims all along the highways of life. These victims often suffer from anxiety which is another cause of stress. Stress can come in many other forms including demands at work or school.

In the pursuit of dreams, we can enjoy the ride, but we must not fail to contemplate the potential for a setback or failure. It is wise to listen carefully, and then observe what is shown you in order to remember what is important. From years of experience, it seems the dental chair or doctor's office can erase or block people's ability to remember. So, try to be alert and calm so you can ask the right questions, even if your perception is blurred by fear or confusion. And remember just because a procedure worked or did not work with a friend or a brother or sister does not mean you will get the same result. This is often the case in orthodontics where front teeth must be rotated or moved in the mouth of an adult. An older person may lose the thin bone around the front side of roots leading to recession, sensitivity and poor cosmetics. Adults must take care when sharing simple warnings like, "it will only hurt a little," with children. It can be magnified in a child's mind leading to uncontrollable fear.

Appropriate positive thoughts and concern. Listen and learn. Prevent disasters by applying what you learn to establish good habits. A very significant problem Dr. Hofmann sees in the mouth is caused by brushing incorrectly. Too hard a toothbrush bristle, or too much pressure can cut deep grooves and "beaver-like" cuts into the roots and enamel of teeth. This can happen to anyone who uses an ultrasonic toothbrush too aggressively. At one time companies promoted these hyper-toothbrushes for the handicapped. Unfortunately, this is a good way to destroy teeth. Large grain baking soda or salt can also create severe damage to enamel, dentin, and bone. They are too abrasive and anti-bacterial, and you want to preserve good bacteria. Wrong thinking can really harm your mouth and health.

Some people think the more they brush their teeth the whiter their teeth will become. Wrong, just the opposite is true. Once you remove the enamel the darker dentin will start to show through. This is a reminder that some home remedies and myths may be dangerous. Read the Chapter on "Myths" to discover answers to other misconceptions concerning your mouth and teeth.

Obsessive brushing can be more destructive than tooth decay! Brush gently, at a 45-degree angle to the gingival (gum) collar and use a mild toothpaste. To clean the backside of the far back molars use a small headed brush and close your teeth together while pulling the cheek back. Remove food stuck on teeth so it will not harden into a rock-hard calcium carbonate called calculus. These thorn-like deposits irritate the tissue and allow bacteria to hide around teeth, destroying bone and causing pockets. It allows bacteria to acidify the area and prevents good saliva, mouth rinses, floss, and a toothbrush from healing tissue.

This is Periodontal disease and next to tooth decay it is the most prevalent disease in the world and the major cause of tooth loss in adults. It is a chronic disease that can produce cell damaging enzymes which are then carried in your blood to many organs in the human body including the heart, lungs, brain and pancreas. Therefore, it is very important to cultivate a healthy saliva by learning techniques and methods to control bad bacteria.

Another area of damage can be done by the unconscious grinding of teeth. Remember when you chew there is food or chewing gum between your teeth. The enamel is not abraded and therefore, is not worn down. However, when you grind during the night while sleeping or grit during the day there is blunt, abrasive tooth-to-tooth contact all the time which will destroy cusps, fillings, veneers, and even crowns! Chewing ice can also be very destructive. Slow down and ease up on the caffeine. The conscious gripping or clenching of your teeth is so destructive it can cause fillings to pop off or break. Likewise, it can also crack teeth, porcelain on crowns, denture teeth, bridge connections, and other structures in the mouth. It will also aggravate bone loss especially if you have periodontal disease. Grinding will move a loose tooth back and forth destroying the thin bone at the neck.

Clinching is different than grinding, and it also can destroy teeth. Clenching or grasping objects with your front teeth can microscopically bend your front teeth to the point where fillings on curved surfaces will pop out or loosen up.

This is because teeth have a different coefficient of flexibility than fillings. And do not open any sealed bags with your teeth. Along with the forces of grinding these micro-movements may aid in the erosion at the necks of teeth.

If you clench during the day, wear a day-guard made of soft plastic or when that is not possible, chew on xylitol gum. If you have porcelain crowns on your upper teeth, be aware grinding or clenching can easily destroy lower natural teeth. Dr. Hofmann sees this type of excessive wear when people have their upper front teeth crowned with porcelain for cosmetic purposes and do nothing to protect weaker lower tooth enamel.

This is a common error in dentistry. Below is an example showing teeth that have lost 70% of their original length. The destruction is on the front and top of her lower front teeth and the circular markings you see are the calcified root channels where the nerve used to be: almost all the enamel is gone - Figure 6.

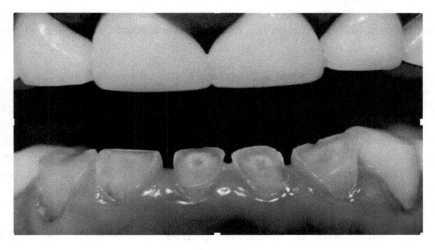

Many professionals believe that stress can generate the formation of calculus or calcium carbonate which leads to the formation of periodontal disease. Our body acts like a living electromagnet especially during times of stress. Your mouth can become a low-grade battery with acidic calcium-rich saliva. The tooth enamel has a negative charge, which naturally tends to attract positive charged ions such as hydrogen and calcium ions. These calcium ions and anything that makes saliva more acidic can help generate calculus. This may be why adults have much more calculus than children even though everyone in the family is eating the same foods.

The most common area for calculus buildup is behind your lower front teeth since that is where the *sub-lingual* and *sub-mandibular* salivary glands secrete calcium rich saliva. Bacteria live in and around these porous and rough deposits as they multiply next to your now swollen gum tissue. Their acids will destroy protective fibers and bone, causing swelling, bone loss and periodontal disease. When brushing this swollen gum tissue will often bleed.

Bad bacteria in *plaque* will concentrate bad acids wherever they adhere to teeth and tissue. A good example is the streptococcus bacteria which is a cause of strep throat. The 5-carbon sugar-alcohol, xylitol can counter the production of these acids by preventing the bad bacteria from metabolizing 6-carbon sugars such as sucrose or fructose. By decreasing acids, xylitol can help decrease decay and the formation of calculus. Research is showing that xylitol can also disrupt *Pseudomonas aeruginosa*, another deadly bacterium hiding in debris around teeth. Like *Strep mutans* these bad bacteria are opportunistic and can cause serious problems such as pneumonia. There is more information on this dynamic balance and "saliva war" in coming chapters.

The mouth is a key organ for measuring general health. Since the tongue is so vascular our mouth is a good barometer of what is going on throughout the body. *Mucosal* cells in the mouth grow and die faster than most other cells in the body. These cells are more susceptible to irritation. The tooth on the other hand has the toughest structural material in the body and amazingly it can also be destroyed by acids from bacteria. What we eat, breathe, and drink through our mouth is key to protecting and maintaining these tissues and organs. Therefore, it is important to end those bad habits that are deeply ingrained in our pleasure centers and replace them with good habits and foods.

More than 25% of Dr. Hofmann's patients have partially destroyed their teeth due to over-brushing, grinding or acid erosion. Some of this acid erosion is from acid reflux, carbonated sodas, energy drinks or juices. He warns people not to suck on lemons, limes or lozenges. Instead use xylitol mints or gum which will neutralize acids. This is especially useful when traveling or at work. If you cannot brush your teeth, xylitol will help. It can also protect nasal passages from airline vent air, bacterial dust, and bacterial aerosols. To those who suffer constipation while traveling, it will loosen your stools and decrease nasal congestion. Take a mint right after a meal or when the acid content of saliva is at its highest which is usually early morning or right before bedtime

Dr. Hofmann testifies, "if I had known this information 40 years ago, xylitol could have rescued me from days of painful sore throats, running noses, missed sleep, and wasted antibiotics. And who knows how those antibiotics affected my gut and my general health?" Amazingly, it is also very effective against infections of the middle ear. As stated earlier this was discovered in the Finnish studies and by many physicians who have used it on children. Note that is best to use a flavor other than mint on children.

Xylitol has the innate ability to help defeat bacteria in many parts of the body while building up bone strength and neutralizing acids in our saliva. It works up and down our body and inside and outside of cells and tissues! It helps defeat a hacking cough, sinus infections and *Candida Albicans* - a pervasive yeast that can invade mucosal tissues in the mouth, throat and colon. Research shows that it also helps ease the effect of cystic fibrosis, and can prevent glaucoma by releasing intra-ocular pressures. A good list of fibrosis studies on xylitol can be found by referencing NIH research and Cystic Fibrosis by Joseph Zabner, completed on February 2015, at Children's Hospital of Chicago.

In conclusion, Dr. Hofmann asks, "Why is xylitol's curing effect not promoted here by the media nor the government? Why do we ignore what many other nations have discovered? As stated, the EU's version of the FDA recognizes the powerful preventive and curative power of xylitol. Is our neglect due to greed or blindness to truth? We spend more money per capita on healthcare than the rest of the world. Little nations like Finland seem to have much lower disease rates with much less capital invested. In contrast our system produces a very profitable drug, alcohol and sugar industry with its extensive and very lucrative retail medicine, hospital-nursing-care and medical-dental professions.

These questions need to be answered before we end up manufacturing a whole population of chronic diseases including dementia, diabetes, Lupus, and other auto-immune disorders. Would it hurt our economy to cut back on both the 6-carbon sugars and artificial sweeteners? It is estimated that income from Halloween candies alone will total over 2.4 billion dollars this year alone. There is a lot of money to be made in the perpetuation of disease, bad diets and drug use. Can we as consumers allow this vicious cycle to get any worse? The best solution is to promote a fiber-nutritive diet and food medicines like xylitol.

CHAPTER NINE
"DOC, I DIDN'T KNOW THAT!"

Dr. Hofmann confides, *"The most important thing I am doing for my patients as a doctor is educating and motivating them to practice safe and effective preventive care! Knowledgeable patients will then have the tools to prevent or stop disease. This philosophy could transform our healthcare."*

<u>Truth-Bites To Save Your Teeth, Your Wallet & Your Life:</u>

1)   Saliva is extremely important for the health of your mouth. It does many things including; washing away food debris that would otherwise contribute to tooth decay and gum disease; initiates a digestive process in the mouth; and is the solvent which allows for the sensation of taste and the enjoyment of food. People with little saliva or with what scientists call "xerostomia" exhibit signs and symptoms which range from mild to severe oral discomfort and disease. Saliva also protects oral tissue from the friction of jaw and tongue movements and from potential injuries caused by trauma such as biting your cheek. It protects mucosa from the burning heat of a slice of hot pizza and from viral lesions or ulcers. A healthy saliva varies in pH during the day but has an average pH between 6.4 and 7.3 so it can neutralize or buffer acids that erode and demineralize teeth. It also   has immune components which can stave off bacteria, viruses and fungi. These are good reasons not to smoke, vape, or use e-cigs since good cells in saliva will be negatively affected or destroyed. There is more important information about saliva in Chapter 23.

2)   The new ceramic or Zirconia crowns are incredibly strong and will not wear down or break like gold or porcelain crowns. They are cosmetic and kind to opposing teeth. This innovation allows a dentist to make strong crowns in tight places where pressures are high.

3)   Three of the major causes of death are related to the mouth. These are as follows: a) Enzymes from bad bacteria located deep in diseased boney pockets get into the blood stream and can weaken the heart and other organs; b) A weakened heart fails due to oxygen deprivation after bouts of sleep apnea and sleepless nights; and, c) Gram-negative pneumonia spreads into the lungs of the bedridden patient as bacterial plaque falls off unclean teeth and is inhaled.

4)   Oral Cancer is NOT caused by alcohol in Listerine according to Oral Pathologists. Most of us are misinformed. When Pathologists say alcohol is directly related to oral cancer, they are referring to brewed or aged alcohol. The drink you buy at a bar may have carcinogens. The point is alcoholic beverages do not state ingredients nor additives. There may be trace elements pesticides, acetaldehydes, urethans and other chemicals contaminating their secret formula? The fermentation process may absorb contaminants from new wood used in barrels. According to the ADA oral cancer afflicts over 83,000 people a year and on average one person dies each hour in the United States. Note the HPV (Human Papilloma Virus) is a major cause of throat cancer in the sexually active.

5)   Your teeth do not touch when chewing and therefore the wear rate of enamel during chewing is very low. The forces that cause wear are called "parafunctional" forces which are related to grinding or clenching of the teeth. Chewing ice or hard foods and candies, however, can break or erode teeth.

6)   Healthy tooth enamel can stand strong forces due to a micro-structure attachment to dentin. Craze lines or micro-fractures in enamel should not be a big reason for concern. Over time they can develop into a crack which may cause the tooth to break. Clinching is also bad for enamel. The enamel is translucent and if a tooth dies it can turn black. The reason for this is iron particles from the dried blood that once flowed in the tooth are now trapped in the canal. The blood cells and other tissues have dissolved away leaving the iron behind.

7)   Most dental professionals agree fluoride in water has been one of the most effective methods of decreasing the prevalence of tooth decay. City water often has less fluoride than well or aquifer water. Recently Juneau, Alaska made the mistake of stopping fluoridation in its city water and saw the rates of tooth decay rise dramatically among its children.

8)   Yellow tooth enamel can be whitened by oxidizing enamel. Oxygen radicals are attracted to stains in the inter-prismatic spaces within the layers of enamel and then work to bleach the offending color out. After a tooth whitening, light will reflect better in those oxidized prismatic layers. Dr. Hofmann doesn't recommend any fast whitening procedures on young or sensitive teeth. Whitening agents used over a long term can lead to loss of good biofilmand demineralization of enamel and dentin.

9)   Teeth can spontaneously die. A hard impact or calcium build-up inside teeth can kill them. Both fractures and decay can also kill teeth. However, a dead tooth can be saved and restored with a root-canal and crown. The root-canal replaces necrotic tissue with a safe inert filler called gutta percha. And, "NO" root canals do not poison people

nor does crown cement! According to some reports, 19-out-of-20 people having a root canal will have no problems and the tooth will be saved. Older people's teeth can appear grayish. This may be due to their blood becoming bluer in color as the blood becomes less oxygenated.

10) Often patients who are weakened by radiation therapy and cancer have a very low immune response. This is a very good reason to have a loose or highly infected tooth extracted. Also, if you had recent joint surgery remember to take antibiotics prior to a tooth cleaning.

11) Xylitol: a 5-carbon polyol that can heal infection in the mouth and nose by preventing acid-producing bacteria from gaining control. It works well against bad bacteria keeping them from adhering to and penetrating cell layers in the mucosa of the mouth and nasal passages, and from demineralizing enamel and dentin. Unlike the popular nasal saline lavages, it is less likely to harm the healthy mucous and microbiome. Xylitol in spray form tamed Dr. Hofmann's hacking cough and prevented an annual Strep throat bout. In the past when a dry cough started Dr. Hofmann would take a regimen of penicillin. However, it is better to avoid overuse of all antibiotics.

12) Simply rinsing your mouth with the water at your dining table helps to neutralize food and acids in and around teeth. A vigorous flushing may also help dislodge heavier plaque from around teeth. Then just swallow the water.

13) Rotated or leaning teeth can be food-traps, and so it is good to straighten teeth by wearing braces. When you lose a tooth the tooth behind it may start leaning towards the empty space and the tooth above may move downward. As it moves more root surfaces and food traps are exposed. Therefore, it is important to quickly replace the missing tooth with an implant, bridge or a denture tooth attached to a partial denture.

14) Dark chocolate and red wine have polyphenols that are good for the heart and can counter bad "free-radicals" and help prebiotics. Six carbon sugar in any of these products, however, can feed bad bacteria and motivate tooth decay.

15) Xylitol is a natural sugar found both in your body and in plants. It is anti-bacterial, stimulates saliva production, remineralizers your enamel and helps strengthen your bone! Like a 1-2-3 punch it inactivates the bad bacteria and detaches them from their tissue surface or habitat. Then it stimulates the

flow of saliva or other extracellular fluids which washes the bacteria away and neutralizes their acids and toxins. Chewing gum with xylitol improves your saliva by reducing acids and bacteria while helping to clean your teeth! It would be wise to replace some of your table sugar and sugar substitutes with xylitol and use up to 5 grams or one teaspoon three times per day. It will protect the healthy microbiome all the way to the colon.

16)	Swishing	of	acids such as orange juice, or carbonated	drinks is extremely destructive to enamel, for it removes the protective "film layer" that protects the enamel, allowing the enamel to be decalcified. Energy drinks, lozenges, antacids like TUMS and vaping are also potential problems for teeth.

17)	Tooth enamel ranks 4th on a Brinell scale of hardness which is equal to the semi-precious stone Topaz, yet its structure is 4% water.

18)	Many toothpastes have flavorings which can cause burning sensations in the mouth of allergic patients. Another chemical that can cause irritation is sodium lauryl sulfate. This may happen with pre-menopausal women or patients with a dry mouth. A good toothpaste neutralizes acids, cleanses teeth, and helps with tooth remineralization. A good xylitol toothpaste does all three including the stimulation of salivary flow. If you have tooth decay or have had radiation therapy, it is wise to use a extra-fluoridated toothpaste with 2000 times the power of normal toothpaste.

19)	Use a mouth rinse that is not too acidic. Stabilized or activated chlorine dioxide has a more neutral pH, is effective in controlling mouth odors and acts as a soothing disinfectant even in a dry mouth. Most commercial mouth rinses are acidic. Some are so acidic their pH is as low as citric acid.

20)	Bite-wing x-rays are taken once a year so the dentist can check for decay and bone loss between teeth. When you have a toothache, the dentist will usually take a Periapical x-ray of the whole tooth in order to check for an abscess. A Panorex scanning x-ray or full set of x-rays is usually taken every 5-7 years. Digital x-rays use 6 times less radiation than the old celluloid type and are accurate and simple to take.

21)	Why is an exam necessary? We check for cancer, tooth decay, and potential problems. This dental exam is the basis of a legal document.

22)	When moving take your dental records. This is one reason why digital x-rays are better. You can have them sent by email to any part of the world. They can be compared with new ones to check for bone loss. The digital x-ray was developed by the Navy in order to transfer x-rays between ship and shore.

23) Free radicals and acrylamides found in highly heated foods such potato chips brought fear to health-conscious people the world over. We are now beginning to understand another threat, AGE's or Accumulation of Glycation-End products. As the pancreas wears down and unused sugars fail to convert into energy or fat, they bind with and damage proteins. They form glycation products which block small vessels in the heart, brain, eyes, kidneys, and even limbs causing cell and tissue failure.

24) Did you know false ears and noses are made by the Prosthetic dentist? "Yes," this branch of dentistry helps cancer patients and others look normal in public. The dentist is the "master" of impression taking and may be the artist-sculptor who will design and color the prosthetic shape for the face.

25) Many new dental products take time to reach the average dental office. It takes time for dentists to learn and feel comfortable using them. One of these revolutionary new products is silver diamine fluoride or SDF. It can neutralize even deep tooth decay and in many cases no needle nor high-speed drill is required. Other products are xylitol and zinc containing products. You can go to the website: DentistryXposed.com. For updates on research, products, & information. There are also many informative blog posts.

26) A dry mouth and throat can be caused by mouth breathing, medications or nasal congestion. Using a xylitol spray with essential oils in the nasal passages or in the mouth will help control bad bacteria, congestion and inflammation.

27) If you wear a night guard, it is wise to clean your teeth first and then rinse with fluoride before bedtime. Saliva at night and early in the morning is more acidic. This is one reason to finish your eating at night with protein or foods with calcium or phosphate such as cheese, broccoli, yogurt, salty nuts, and avocado. Or gently chew xylitol mints and gum.

28) Teeth are not directly attached to bone, instead thousands of ligaments hold the tooth onto the bone socket. This allows the tooth to "bounce" and not crack when impacted. However, when a tooth is over-stressed it can feel sensitive in much the same way as a sprained ankle. Reducing high spots where the tooth is hitting hard will allow it to heal and prevent death of the tooth or a fracture.

29)   Eating fibrous foods not only helps to cleanse your teeth and decrease the quick intake of sugar, but it can protect the microbiome in the gut and like xylitol they are often converted into a cancer-preventing butyrate in the colon. These prebiotics help the microbiome break down the nutrients that keep you healthy. Some examples are: Chicory Root, artichoke, apple skins, garlic, onions, leek, asparagus, walnuts, pistachios, bananas, oat, barley and wheat bran. It has been proven that polyphenols such as chocolate and red wine among many others work to help prebiotics work more effectively.

30)   Chronic inflammation can affect your joints, your energy level and healthy cells throughout the body. It often originates in the gut where the opportunistic yeast *Candida Albicans* multiplies increasing the potential for cancer and aiding in *leaky gut syndrome*. Leaky gut allows foreign proteins and microbes into the bloodstream. Research explained in *Nutrition in Clinical Practice* and in the studies by Dr. Steven Gundry, indicates that a good diet is very important for healthy organs. Every cell needs good nutrients. This process can affect the immune system, body weight, cellular metabolism, and every organ or tissue. He warns that lectins play a big part in a leaky gut and therefore, suggests that people cut down on peanuts, tomatoes, corn, rough grains, poorly cooked beans, cashews, sweeteners such as Splenda and the over use of antibiotics, painkillers, anti-depressants, steroids, anti-inflammatory medications and many other drugs. If your digestion is disrupted and the symbiotic balance of good bacteria is affected, Candida yeast can burrow into the gut lining and cause a leaky gut.

There are a lot of good fiber rich prebiotics that can help probiotics preserve a good balance of bacteria. They can also stop the dangerous yeast *Candida Albicans* and prevent a leaky gut. A safe diet combination is fiber-rich and protein-rich foods with xylitol. If you are taking one of many common medications, it is a good idea to eat probiotic foods like yogurt or if you are lactate intolerant, take a probiotic capsule. There are other good food-medicines besides xylitol; one is turmeric. Turmeric helps both the joints and gut while working against inflammation. Inflammation is a major cause of discomfort and breakdown of healthy tissue. Turmeric will help you cut down on the use of ibuprofen or aspirin, both of which harm the microbiome and aggravate the leaky gut syndrome. One good food idea is a nutritious smoothie made by blending spinach, yogurt, a banana, protein powder, blueberries or raspberries, turmeric, xylitol, ice, and strawberries.

CHAPTER TEN
Emergencies and the Rescue

This may be one of the most important chapters in the book since we never know when the next emergency will happen. As Dr. Hofmann explains it, "Too many times I have heard the common refrain in the middle of the night, 'Doc, I have a bad toothache, can you see me!' In my early days in dentistry, I would say, 'Yes, can you meet me in an hour?'" At that time, he was charged with running the Dental Emergency Services for the local Dental Society. He performed many root canals, denture extractions, repairs on dentures. What he learned may help you in your time of need.

This is one reason why he discovered and trademarked a repair material which would solve the need for a temporary strong repair. It worked well with decayed baby teeth that were soon to be lost. This material was biocompatible and hydrophilic (water-friendly). Since our bodies are over 70% water many materials that are water-friendly are safe and effective in the mouth. It worked well despite an area being contaminated by both saliva and blood and hence it could work well in deep areas where other materials failed to seal or stick. Now we have a new material called SDF or silver diamine fluoride which can eat away decay in deep or tight areas that are hard to get to. It can provide a good foundation for adhesive tooth colored glass-ionomer fillings.

Ironically, on his first mission trip to Africa, he broke his own tooth in the worse place possible, leaving a sharp razor edge next to the leading edge of his tongue. This was a month-long trip to the Gola tribe in the jungles of Liberia and to the ELWA hospital in Monrovia, Liberia (the same hospital which was central in the fight against Ebola during the recent epidemic). His assistant mixed up the "Rescue and Restore" material and placed it into the hole or cavity with a simple instrument.

The material stuck to the old metal filling, the very smooth sharp enamel, and the moist dentin. It relieved his sore tongue and he was finally able to talk and eat normally without discomfort. Even though one fourth of the inside wall of the tooth had sheared off in the main chewing area, this temporary held on for the entire trip! Later, using a Swiss army knife and glass slat, he repaired a missionary's tooth that had a missing metal filling.

Rescue and Restore worked well repairing teeth of those patients who broke a tooth or a filling while traveling through Dallas. One amazing example was an older gentleman who was undergoing chemotherapy and broke one of only two teeth he had on his entire lower jaw. The tooth had a crown-post which broke through the root and prevented him from wearing his lower partial. Dr. Hofmann told him the material was strong, but that it would be a miracle if it lasted more than 10 minutes under the powerful rocking forces created by all the denture teeth on either side pulling or pushing like a seesaw. He said, "Do it anyway." Dr. Hofmann did as he commanded and amazingly it lasted the entire few weeks that he was under cancer treatment in Dallas.

Dentists from the military hospital where he was a patient were so amazed, they asked Dr. Hofmann to explain the formula! When he tried to market the material, lawyers from a major Wall Street Corporation called him up and warned him their extended patent prevented him from merchandising it. He was told that if he attempted to market it, they would sue him.

If you have a sharp edge, the information on the Internet suggests covering it with chewing gum, orthodontic-wax or paraffin wax. It can temporarily block the sharp tooth from the tongue but will not hold long. The best solution is to find a dentist who will smooth over the edge until a more permanent solution such as a filling or crown can be placed. If you have a whitening tray, it can cover a sharp edge while you talk or sleep. Do this only for a short time since the rubbery surface will prevent free movement of your jaw while asleep.

Freedom to glide is good for the health of your jaw-joints and a good reason not to buy an over-the-counter thermoplastic night guard. The plastic in those bulky heat-sensitive night guards is not as hard as a professional heat-sunk night guard. They can distort and aren't comfortable. They can pick up odors and discolor over time since the plastic is part soft thermoplastic.

Dr. Hofmann suggests using special extra-hard ortho-plastic which is heat sunk on a stone model of your teeth: He charges less than $200 for these which is much lower than the average insurance charge of $350. He does this in order to motivate people not to delay. These are very comfortable and last for years, unless you step on it or let your pet dog or cat eat it. The night guard will protect teeth from wear, stabilizing them from harmful stresses.

He has one more solution for the sharp edge of a cracked tooth. It is the glass nail file made in Czech Republic and available at Walmart & H-Mart. BE CAREFUL and DO THIS ONLY IF YOU ARE GOOD WITH YOUR HANDS.

With gentle care use the file to smooth the razor-sharp edge of the enamel. This type of nail file never wears out and can be used to smooth over fillings or enamel which feel rough or sharp. This advice can save you a lot of money and prevent pain and discomfort. It helped Dr. Hofmann, recently when he broke a cusp off. Then see your dentist as soon as you can for repairs.

Some decayed teeth have a different kind of fracture which is like an eggshell breaking. When the enamel collapses a crater-type hole forms on top of the tooth. This happens when deep decay penetrates the enamel and undermines it. Do not try to place a temporary in this kind of hole, as this will only cover decay, and prevent the good saliva from neutralizing bacteria and acids. The hole in a cratered tooth might be acting as a drain for exudate or pus! It may also act as an escape for toxic gases which build up inside an infected tooth's pulp chamber and root canals.

If you plug the hole the infection lifts the tooth into the bite due to hydraulic pressures of air and liquid. This increases the pain and might cause tissue to swell. When you bite, it will impact harder and harder, irritating the already sore tooth, causing more and more pain. If you cannot find a dentist, you can use a drop of clove oil to help ease the pain. Dr. Hofmann asked Walmart to stock it and they did. This is good to know. If enough people request it, Walmart may stock xylitol too. Keep some clove oil in your Emergency Kit. When needed put a drop on a small cotton ball and place it in the hole or rub it onto the gum around the tooth with a cotton swab; and see your dentist as soon as possible.

A toothache can be a miserable experience which most people never forget. Also include cotton balls, clove oil, Q-tips, and a mouth mirror in your Emergency kit. If your child cracks a front tooth, keep that broken piece. If a tooth is knocked out of the socket, place the tooth in milk or a saline solution and see the dentist as soon as possible.

As head of the Dallas Dental Society's Emergency Services, Dr. Hofmann often saw many interesting cases including an ex-Cowboy player who came in with his girlfriend and was so scared he asked her to sit with him on the dental treatment chair. Other cases were people looking for drugs. When it comes to pain there are many gray areas that can trip-up a dentist. The dentist must help the patient in pain while at the same time use common sense to determine if the tooth is really the source of pain. Drug users will not treat the tooth that is his "deal-maker." That tooth is often an old root canaled tooth with an unhealed abscess. They will fake pain, and if they make an appointment, they will not show up.

The DEA and State agencies have been very good at regulating the prescription of opioids. But it is up to the dentist to determine what is "real pain." Just to be safe, the dentist should prescribe a low number of opioid-type pills, for the good of the patient. In most states, we can no longer "call in" a controlled painkiller, like hydrocodone. The patient must be seen, and a special script used. This is how the state and federal agencies can monitor the over prescription of narcotics.

A possible addition to your Emergency Dental First Aid kit is a dozen gel-cap 300 mg ibuprofen (for an adult), and a dozen 325 mg. Tylenol. The combination creates a synergy which can potentiate the pain-relieving effects of both. If you are sensitive to either medication or have any complicating condition do not take them. Be aware that too much ibuprofen and other NSAIDs will dry out your mouth and can create a leaky gut. As stated earlier a dry mouth promotes both tooth decay and periodontal disease. A leaky gut can lead to many other problems including auto-immune and degenerative diseases. It is important for both the medically compromised and elderly to consult with their physician. And note other important contra-indications listed in Chapter 18.

Do good searches on both the internet and in books. One good book is Andrew Weil's book, *Healthy Aging*. Check out Dr. Hofmann's web and blog site called DentistryXposed.com, where you can read good articles and leave comments or reviews. You can also contact him or respond on the Facebook page Dentistry Xposed or the dental website: DentalRescue.com. Other Facebook pages to check out are Peter Hofmann DDS or Smile Dentist USA.

CHAPTER ELEVEN
Myth Busting

Twenty-three Important Answers:

1) It is natural to lose your teeth. This is FALSE: The truth is your teeth should last a lifetime. Unfortunately, we are often lured into a bad diet of sugar and empty carbohydrates. What good is it to have great dental care if we provide poor preventive care? Many people fail to go to a dentist for annual checkups. Some believe life will be easier without teeth, but they need to know two important points: First you will have only 40% of chewing efficiency with false teeth and second you will tend not to eat the green leafy vegetables and other good fibrous foods which are necessary for good health.

2) Eating Cookies and Cake is OK compared to sugar. This is FALSE: The truth is Empty or processed carbohydrates are equal to sugar and maybe worse. Enzymes in your mouth convert these empty calories into sugar. But this sugar compound is glue-like and can form a sticky plaque on tooth surfaces. Bacteria that live in the plaque form destructive acids which cause tooth decay and gum disease. Plaque can harden into a rock-hard substance called calculus which is the main cause of periodontal disease. Bacteria hides under this hardened plaque and destroys fiber, tissue, and bone, causing gums to turn red and swell.

3) All Sugars Are BAD. This is FALSE: There are good sugars such as Xylitol which is a low-caloric sugar-alcohol found naturally in your body, trees and plants. It has 40% less calories than sugar and has very low glycemic index of 7 versus 70 for sugar. It is both anti-bacterial and good for enamel, saliva, and bone. Chewing xylitol mints or chewing xylitol gum is especially good since it improves the quality of saliva, helps with re-mineralization of teeth, and inhibits bad bacteria from harming teeth and mucosa. If you have a xylitol mint or gum after meals or snacks, or 3-5 times per day, it will do a lot to preserve your good bacteria from the mouth down to the colon. The over promotion and sweetening of foods or drink is another sad example of manufactured disease for the sake of profits.

4) The major cause of tooth loss in adults is tooth decay. This is FALSE: Periodontal disease is the main cause of tooth loss in people over the age of 35 with most people having some form of the disease. Ten percent of them have serious gum disease. Gingivitis which is a precursor to the more serious gum disease called periodontal disease, is less destructive. If you eat healthy and take care of your saliva and teeth, you can maintain a healthy disease-free mouth. Acids from drinks, fruit and acid reflux can destroy large areas of enamel on teeth and result in rampant tooth decay or destruction of the bite.

5) Bleeding gums when brushing is normal - FALSE: Bleeding gums is a sign of gingivitis or gum inflammation. Brushing and flossing helps to massage and clean the gums, so they do not bleed. Also going to the dentist regularly to control the hard plaque, called calculus, will help the healing. This is the reason for the dentist scraping your teeth with metal "scalers." Just remember good care leads to quick repair and eventually restored health. If you are pregnant, gums often do swell and bleed more, so do not be alarmed. Just keep them as clean as you can by using a good mouth rinse like activated chlorine dioxide and xylitol chewing gum. Xylitol will control both the bad bacteria and the acids they produce.

6) Root canals will poison you. This is FALSE: This myth is spread by fear mongers some of whom call themselves "holistic." They cause harm by promoting ideas which lead people to make bad decisions. "Yes," some root canals fail because they were done wrong by the operator but that is also very true of crowns and bridges done by many dentists. Inflammation around a crown can be more dangerous than an abscess.

Dentists make a lot of money off crowns. Teeth are unique in that they have a very hard outer matrix called enamel which protects the nerves in the pulp. If infected the inner chamber needs to be sterilized and cleaned out, then sealed with an inert material called "gutta percha." Once the canal or canals are sealed properly the lesion or abscess will normally heal on its own and the tooth will function as a normal tooth. Since root canaled teeth are no longer alive, they can become brittle. This is a good reason to crown them. We should do everything possible to save teeth. A missing tooth can cause extensive problems including the drifting of any tooth that once contacted it. Root canals also allow us to save the original bone around a tooth. Extracting a tooth allows the bone to dissolve away creating a defect in the bone that can look unattractive in the front or be a food trap in the back.

7) Apple-Cider Vinegar is good for my teeth. This is <u>FALSE</u>: There is a major company that wants to make this acid additive the answer to many ailments in the body. The fact is sipping a few teaspoons in a cup of water can destroy teeth. The problem is people think it is perfectly safe since few warnings are posted. People sip the mix over-and-over again during the day for digestion and other problems. Dr. Hofmann had two of these patients in just a week, each with rampant tooth decay, despite having good oral hygiene and a history of low sugar consumption. Why are warnings not posted in promotions and books? Some ads claim that Apple Cider Vinegar is a pharmacy-in-a-bottle. Thankfully, there is a much more effective food medicine that deserves the honor. Xylitol works top-down from the mouth and nasal passages to the colon preserving a healthy microbiome, and controlling the multiplication and spread of bad bacteria. It helps prevent leaky gut syndrome and colon cancer caused by Candida yeast. Candida Albicans is opportunistic as it awaits a weakened body or poor diet to spread and attack. It loves regular sugar but does not feed on Xylitol.

8) Alcohol causes cancer. This is TRUE & FALSE: Depending on how you define alcohol." Alcohol in Listerine does not cause cancer. Pathologists say alcohol irritation is not a cause of cancer. The cause is cell-wall infiltration by carcinogenic compounds or viruses. Apparently some fermented or distilled alcohols have carcinogenic impurities which penetrate cell walls causing cancer. Scientists suspect aldehyde and other carcinogens may be incorporated in the fermentation or preparation of the drinking alcohol. The drying effect of alcohol along with tobacco smoke can increase the rate and amount of tooth-decay and periodontal disease primarily on upper teeth. This would also be true of smoking marijuana and other products.

Your saliva and a healthy layer of biofilm protect your teeth, bone, and gingival tissue. Do everything possible to protect them, including decreasing acid intake and snacking. The sipping of any drink throughout the day is bad. Let your saliva rest and do not dilute it with constant sipping of any drink.

9) Brushing Teeth is not important. This is FALSE: Brushing with the soft bristles of a properly designed toothbrush and pointing them at a 45-degree angle to the collar is very effective in the proper care of teeth and the gingival tissue. DO NOT apply too much pressure and, if you have erosion only use a super-soft toothbrush. By fighting the bad bacteria, you can decrease bone loss and

the potential release of destructive enzymes into the blood stream.

10) Ultrasonic brushes are always safe - FALSE: You must use the gentle mode with soft bristles. It should be noted that the misuse of ultrasonic brushes can cause a lot of damage. Dr. Hofmann believes these devices are oversold without proper warnings needed to prevent stripping of gum tissue. The ultra-sonic bristles are much stiffer and harder than a good super-soft toothbrush.

11) If I do not have pain, my tooth must be OK. This is FALSE: The fact is many bad problems in the mouth will not cause pain until it is too late to restore the tooth easily. Try to repair your teeth before you need a root canal. One reason people do not feel an obvious warning pain is that decay between teeth keeps food and cold water out. Pain may not happen if the infection does not buildup pressure. If you do have an initial pain, go and see your dentist and have an x-ray taken. Usually periodontal disease is a painless disease, yet it can destroy a lot of bone and tissue. Bone loss would normally freak you out.

12) It is good to brush with salt or regular baking soda. This is FALSE: Both are very abrasive and can cause both erosion and recession on gum tissue, enamel, and dentin. If you have "beaver cuts" on the roots of your teeth, this may be caused by an abrasive toothpaste, acids, or a hard-bristled brush. Also, too much pressure on brushing for too long a time can cause this wear. Chemicals such as citric acid from lemons can decalcify tooth enamel. Gastric acids can also eat away the teeth. Never swish with coke, apple cider vinegar, or orange juice. When you swish you are removing a protective film-layer. This film layer or biofilm helps to protect your tooth from acids and their ability to decalcify teeth.

13) The harder the brush the better it cleans. This is FALSE: As indicated in the above numbers 9 & 12, hard toothbrushes will cause erosion on teeth and can harm the gum tissue. Imagine a large shoe brush and how important it is for the bristles to be soft as you brush and polish around the curves. As the bristles bend, they reach gently into curved and open spaces between teeth and into the 3mm gum collar around the teeth, massaging and cleaning these delicate areas.

16) My parents had dentures; therefore, I will lose my teeth - FALSE: Unfortunately, some young people want all their teeth pulled in the belief it will save them a lot of future trouble and money. Dr. Hofmann refused to pull or extract many teeth in his career because the tooth was in too good a condition to remove. Keeping two strategically located teeth can make a denture very stable. If you plan to have a partial denture instead of implants, save your teeth, especially in the lower jaw where a complete denture gives you only 30% of your normal chewing efficiency. The partial will at least double that efficiency. Your natural teeth will add greatly to good health.

15) Once I pull all my teeth I never have to worry about infections - FALSE: Many serious infections happen underneath full and partial dentures when people fail to remove them at night or just do not clean them. Fungal, yeast, and bacterial infections can cause changes in the gingival tissue which may require surgery to correct.

16) My molar bridge is so good I do not need to clean underneath it - FALSE You must clean under your bridge to both remove food and massage the tissue. Super-floss soaked in stannous fluoride, chlorhexidine or the stabilized chlorine dioxide work well to neutralize the bad bacteria.

17) I will always have sensitive teeth. The TRUTH is as we grow older teeth become more calcified and less sensitive. When you are young your pulp chamber and nerve canals are very large, and so slight drilling on teeth can be felt. Many people only remember the pain they had as a child. You will be surprised how less sensitive adult teeth are. Do not be afraid. The nerve channels and chamber shrink as calcium is laid down, helping to make teeth less sensitive. In many cases older patients do not need anesthetic when having fillings. One good way to erase sensitivity is to get a cotton roll and break off a wad of cotton. Then saturate it in stannous fluoride and press it up against the sensitive area before you go to bed. Do this for a week and the sensitivity should go away.

18) Soap is bad for teeth. This is FALSE: Soap products are often very good and safe at killing bacteria. That is why we use the liquid soap called chlorhexidine to kill bacteria. It is one of the few safe substances which kills both gram positive

and negative bacteria and their spores. Soap will leave a soap scum that continues to kill like a time capsule, but it can also leave a stain. Therefore, target its use for specific areas. This stain can be removed when you have your teeth cleaned. It also works to control odor in the mouth and works well in areas of deep bone loss. If you find yourself without toothpaste you can brush with soap. It kills bad bacteria without hurting human cells.

19) Crowns are always good for teeth. This is FALSE: A correctly constructed crown is good and has many functions including protecting the tooth from fracture and improving the cosmetics. However, many crowns are poorly cemented or do not fit the shape and contour of natural teeth. These artificial teeth can act as food traps and draw food to crown margin areas which are sensitive to tooth decay. Dr. Hofmann believes the fewer the crowns the better. Porcelain crowns cause severe wear against natural teeth and therefore should only be used against porcelain.

20) High Fructose Corn syrup is safe and will not cause tooth decay. This is FALSE: A study in 2013 showed High Fructose Corn Syrup can contribute to tooth decay by pulling good minerals away from teeth and bones. Losing those minerals can weaken the tooth leaving them open to decay. It also adds unnatural amounts of fructose which is easily converted into fat leading to obesity or fatty liver disease. This can lead to insulin resistant diabetes. HFCS must be metabolized in the liver where it forms AGE's or Accumulated Glycation End-products. AGE's can affect many organs as it clogs capillaries in various tissues. HFCS is found in most sweet drinks including teas, sports drinks, sodas, juices and in many candies and yogurt. It is also found in Ketchup, applesauce, pickles, pretzels, jams, peanut butter, nutrition bars, mayonnaise, salad dressing, fruit cups, cereals and many other packaged foods.

21) Amalgams already in the mouth will poison me - FALSE: A seasoned amalgam is a stable metal alloy which does not emit mercury nor any other poison when chewing. Amalgam is safe and accepted by the American Dental Association. Amalgam is composed of a silver-copper-tin mix and some believe amalgam alloy can inhibit the growth of bacteria in tooth decay. We do know that the treated silver in SDF works to stop decay. The removal of zinc and the addition of copper has made amalgam fillings safer and stronger. The tensile strength of amalgam can be 2-4 times greater than tooth colored fillings. This is why it is a very good solution for men or anyone with more jaw muscle power. When a cavity is between teeth it requires extra strength to bridge the gap from the cavity to the edge of the next tooth. Amalgams can handle the impact and will also resist wear better. Tooth colored fillings bowl-out exposing the walls or cusps of the the tooth to fracture.

22) A water jet is an effective way to remove food from between teeth: This is NOT ALWAYS TRUE. In a healthy mouth the gingival papilla that seals the inter-dental area (between teeth) will repel the water jet. Water will just bounce off this tissue and will not penetrate between the teeth. However, if you have bone loss and the spaces are open with the papilla receded, the water-jet can help. It can also work well around implants, under bridges, under and around fixed retainers and some other hard to get areas. The remote battery version can be used to clean teeth in a shower area. You can also blend fluoride or activated chlorine dioxide with water in it's reservoir tank.

23) I can always trust textbooks. This is FALSE: Textbooks show the anatomy of the human tongue mapped out with zones for taste. They falsely teach the tongue has sour taste buds only in back. This was shown not to be true in the 70's. Yet it stayed in textbooks for decades. This is a weakness in our system.

24) Stevia is perfectly safe. This is FALSE: some studies show that Stevia has a negative impact on blood pressure, liver, kidney, heart, hormone activity and the microbiome. It can also adversely affect steroid and cancer medications. High dosage or long use can also affect pregnancy conditions by increasing the workload on heart, kidney and bladder.

A good protection for the microbiome is a high protein, low sugar and heavy fiber diet. This diet is also effective in stopping the yeast Candida and preventing gum diseases. Diets that are high in sugar, simple carbs, and fat will encourage the growth of Candida and other bad microbes that are efficient at extracting the energy from food. Some believe that this process may also tell the body to store energy as fat. And some studies show that both diabetes and obesity may be linked to periodontal disease. Thus, if you include diabetes and oral cancer with the other 3 other mouth connected diseases mentioned earlier, one could easily make the case that 5 of the top 10 causes of death in America are related to the mouth.

Eventually we will develop scientifically designed diets based on each person's DNA that will help defeat obesity, diabetes, auto-immune disorders along with many chronic and acute diseases. This will be possible with the use of pharmacogenomic testing of our saliva. This saliva testing can also help prevent drug overdosing, allergic reactions to prescribed drugs, and other problems such as "drug fog" caused by both drug interactions and overuse.

CHAPTER TWELVE
<u>Knowing Basic</u>

TERMINOLOGY

General Dentistry and Specialties in the field of Dentistry:

A General Dentist does everything including root canals, dentures, extractions, implants, bridges, tooth cleaning and bleaching, fillings, Cosmetic Crowns and veneers, night guards, braces, space-maintainers, and other appliances. They should refer tough cases to the one of the specialists below:

Endodontist: is a specialist of the root structure and performs root canals. They perform very difficult root canals and any surgery related to disease, degeneration, or fracture of the roots. They often work with special microscopes to navigate the narrow canals of roots.

Oral Surgeons: is a specialist in the removal of teeth, tumors, cancer, exostosis and other growths. They also place implants and do major surgery on the TMJ, maxilla, and jaw reconstruction.

Orthodontists: Specializes in placing braces and any device used to straighten teeth. Pediatric Dentist: Specializes in dentistry for children and teens.

Periodontist: is a specialist that focuses on the health of the gingiva, bone, and tooth matrix. They are concerned with function, form, prevention, and esthetics. They grow bone and graft both bone and fibrous gingival tissue to restore health and create an appealing look.

Prosthodontist: specializes in the reconstruction of the teeth for both function and cosmetics. They are often needed for full mouth reconstruction of the mouth and often place implants. They also make implant retained dentures.

Terminology as a Steppingstone to Google Searches:

Synonyms:

Cavity = Tooth Decay.
Calculus = Tartar = Rock-Like buildup on teeth.
Prophylaxis = Prophy = Cleaning of Teeth
Crowns = Caps, and 3 or more crown units fused together = a Bridge.
Doctor = both dentists and physicians.
Deep Cleaning = Scaling & Root Planning
Gingiva = Gums = Soft tissue around teeth. Calculus = tartar = hardened plaque, which consists of food, bacteria, dead cells, and other particles.

The following definitions are simple explanations and are not scientifically detailed definitions. For instance, "Crowns" are placed to protect the surfaces of teeth, and thus can be used to change the color and shape of the tooth.

3/4 Crown leaves the cosmetic outside wall of a tooth's enamel alone to save tooth structure and to give the tooth a more natural look.

3-Unit Bridge is a bridge composed of 3 adjoining crown units. It typically has two abutments and one middle pontic that links or bridges the two crowns or abutments. Can be placed on teeth or implants.

All-on-4 implant restoration is a way to restore an entire arch of teeth with just four implants and a zirconia bridge-like span of teeth in the arch.

Amalgam or Silver Filling is a combination of powdered silver, zinc, copper, tin and liquid mercury. All are mixed (triturated) to form an alloy called amalgam. The filling is strong and long lasting. It can be burnished or shaped to create an ultra-smooth surface. It's contact with enamel, dentin and adjoining teeth is near perfect in smoothness and strength, preventing food and decay from collecting. *Amalgamation* is the process from mixing to hardening.

Amylase is the enzyme in the saliva that helps to digest carbohydrates by converting starch into sugar. This process does create a sticky paste-like plaque which will attach to teeth.

Anaerobic bacteria are bad bacteria which do not live on oxygen but live deep in gum and bone defects and are responsible for gum and bone loss.

Anecdotal account is a record of a patient's or doctor's experience with conclusions in matters of a successful treatment or care.

Biofilm is a slimy buildup of bacteria that forms on the surfaces of teeth.

Bite-wing x-rays scans upper and lower back teeth at crown level only. They do not include the roots of the teeth but are good at detecting decay and bone loss.

Bone Growth Stimulants such as Emdogain, work to regenerate bone that is against a tooth or implant.

Bowling-out effect explains the bowl-shaped wear created by an opposing cusp as it cuts into a large white filling. It can cause the collapse of the bite which in turn causes severe wear of the front teeth and therefore a cosmetic issue.

BPA is a type of plastic once used for water bottles. It may contribute to the neurological development problems in children and may lead to cancer formation.

Carcinogens or carcinogenic refers to cancer causing molecules which can also be manufactured naturally or by cooking.

Clear aligners and Fast Braces: Two techniques to straighten teeth that can often be performed by the General dentist and are generally cheaper than traditional orthodontics. Invisalign is a tooth aligner system for teens & adults.

Cementum or cement on the root preserves the root attachment to the bone and the fine fibers at the neck of teeth.

Ceramic Crown: This Ceramic-metal technology is cosmetic in color yet is a form of metal. It is also called Zirconia ceramic and they are extremely strong.

Chlorine Dioxide is effective in oxidizing chemicals which cause malodor and helps eliminate anaerobic bacteria in the mouth.

COPD or Chronic Obstructive Pulmonary Disease, is a lung disease often caused by long term exposure to gases and smoke.

CPAP stands for Continuous Positive Airway Pressure and its accompanying appliance feeds air into your lungs while positioning the jaw forward to open the airway passage. The appliance releases pressure from the tongue, soft palate, and other tissue that can block the airway. Even tonsils or adenoids can be a factor.

Crossbite: is when your lower teeth extend beyond the upper teeth. Normally all upper teeth extend beyond the lower.

Crowns: There are many types of crowns including those made of porcelain, gold, and ceramic. They cover the visible tooth.

Cusp or cusps are the points on a molar tooth, or the pointed prominence on teeth which allow for chewing efficiency.

Dental-dynamic is a word Dr. Hofmann coined to explain all that goes on in the mouth and its interrelationship to good health and function.

Digitial X-rays use 6 X less radiation: therefore are safer. They are easier to copy. Ask the dentist to show you the defect, disease, fracture, or other problem on the x-ray! An x-ray is only two dimensional and so can miss decay. Ask your dentist to compare old with new x-rays.

DNA & RNA have a ribose or pentose sugar in the long strand: DNA stands for Deoxyribonucleic Acid and RNA is **Ribo**nucleic acid and both are key to repair and building of tissues and cells.

Dry Mouth is a condition where Saliva is not being produced by glands and cells resulting in a dry mouth. This condition can also be caused by mouth breathing. People who snore or have sleep apnea may have a dry mouth and more decay on upper and anterior teeth. A dry mouth increases the likelihood for other problems including periodontal disease and rampant tooth decay.

Enamel: Outer layer of teeth which includes the cusps. Loss of the enamel on the top of your teeth will result in vertical loss causing a collapse of your bite –all of which can be prevented by wearing a NIGHTGUARD. The worn-out enamel is easily fractured with hard candy, ice and other objects. Eroded or worn-out enamel is unattractive and can cause sensitivity an ugly smile and facial wrinkles.

Evidence-based Research is based on sound doctor to patient research in the real world of dentistry.

Exudate includes inter-cellular fluids, pus and bacterial-laden fluids with bacteria-fighting cells and cells that have died.

False Pockets vs Periodontal Pockets: This is very important to know, so that you can determine whether you really need a "deep cleaning." More will be discussed on this topic in the "ugly" chapter.

Fibroblast: Cell that initiates healing in the connective tissues around roots of teeth and gingival tissue.

Film Layer is the protective layer over teeth created by saliva that contains bacteria, bacteria-fighting cells, and proteins such as enzymes.

Flora refers to the normal healthy balance of bacteria in the mouth or nose. This flora creates a protective biofilm on the teeth.

Fluoride comes in many forms. In the earth mineral fluorite dissolves in water to form ions . Ground water can have dangerous levels of fluoride which can cause fluorosis of teeth (yellow and white splotches on teeth. Some water systems remove this extra fluoride and other systems add fluoride to a level of .7 parts per million. By law over the counter mouth rinses which say "with fluoride" cannot have more than .7 parts per million. Dentistry now has a powerful new fluoride called SDF or Silver diamine fluoride that will destroy decay. A new toothpaste, Colgate Total SF (SF for Stannous flouride) helps with gum inflammation. Sodium fluoride is commonly used in over-the-counter rinses.

Full denture: Replaces all the teeth in an arch. Partials, and Flippers are removable tooth replacements that replace only some of the teeth. Partials are often made of metal and have cast clasps, whereas flippers typically replace 1-3 teeth, are made of acrylic, and do not have cast clasps. They, however, may have wrought wire clasps which are more flexible and therefore can last longer.

Full Mouth Rebuild or Reconstruction is the best solution for the collapsed bite or what is called "loss of vertical." This involves restoring the occlusion of every tooth to the original length. If teeth are missing then bridges, implants, or partial dentures can be used to restore the bite. This restores vertical loss when the top enamel is eroded.

Furcation is bone loss between two roots of a tooth leaving a pocket in the bone. It is a result of periodontal disease between the roots of molar teeth.

Geriatric: Refers to the elderly or typically those over 80 years of age.

Gingival Collar encircles the tooth with a PDL (Periodontal Ligament and other periodontal fibers) attaching the gingiva to the bone and the bone to the cementum (or the root of the tooth). A Healthy collar is 3 mm. deep and appears pink and firm.

Glass ionomer filling is a type of white filling which is more flexible than composites and are self-adhesive. They, however, are not as strong.

Gram-negative Bacteria: Are anaerobic bacteria (that live without oxygen) deep in tissue and therefore are dangerous (virulent). They can cause pneumonia and destruction of bone in deep pockets such as in a severe periodontal infection.

Gross Debridement is often done when a patient has neglected his or her teeth for a long time and thus requires much more calculus removal, stain removal, and plaque removal. This charge is not covered 100% by insurance like a typical cleaning is.

Gutta Percha points are shaped to fit into a tooth's root canal to seal it off along with a paste sealer. It can also be injected into a root with a heating device which liquefies it for insertion. It is totally non-toxic, natural and safe. It comes from the sap of a tropical tree and with a good sealant prevents bacterial entry.

HPV - Human Papilloma Virus an STD or sexually transmitted disease, may increase the risk of cancer in the throat. Adding to this is the abuse of alcohol, drugs, and all types of smoke. Unfortunately, Dr. Hofmann has known 5 people with oral cancer and none of them were smokers! This runs counter to many studies, but it illustrates that small samples do not represent the general population and can give false conclusions. The ADA records one person per hour dies of oral related cancers. Many of these are throat cancers related to HPV = Human Papilloma Virus. If you have a sore anywhere which is painful and will not go away, see the dentist immediately.

HF Corn Syrup or High Fructose Corn Syrup is found in many popular drinks and foods & is believed to be a major cause of type 2 diabetes.

Hydroxyapatite vs. Fluorapatite crystals utilizes phosphate and calcium. The fluoride ion creates a stronger crystalline structure in enamel.

Implantology is the science of placing implants and restoring them.

Implants are very good replacements for teeth, as they are very strong, highly successful, and can replicate a normal bite. The All-On-Four full arch replacement is very effective and successful for replacement of all the teeth on one arch. Mini implants are smaller and easier to place but have a higher failure rate. They help to retain dentures. Implants do not have ligaments like teeth and therefore impact harder. This impact requires tough crowns like the ceramic or Zirconia crowns.

Incipient decay is minor tooth decay that has not yet penetrated into dentin and so is usually not treated.

Interproximal is an area between two teeth or the surface of each tooth that approximates each other with gum tissue in between.

Ionizing Scans include the 3-D CTscan (Computed Tomography) and the Cone-Beam Computed Tomography scan, or CBCT. Another medical scan is the CAT scan. The MRI is different and does not use any of the ionizing radiation.

Leaky Gut: it is estimated that 80% of the population suffers from increased intestinal permeability which allows bacteria, toxins, & protein molecules to enter the bloodstream.

Male-Female attachment is often a ball and socket type joint used to hold a partial to a root or an implant.

Maxillary Suture line divides the mouth in a symmetrical way from right to left and allows for the growth of the arch.

Media-medicine is another made-up word to emphasize over promotion of archaic and often dangerous concepts and ideas.

Microbiomes are colonies of bacteria growing in colonies which allows for quick production of destructive acids. A good microbiome has less acid production with fewer opportunistic bacteria. Some colonies or microbiome may have hundreds of different bacteria.

MMP8 & MMP9: Matrix metallo-proteinases are a group of zinc-dependent endopeptidases or enzymes which can breakdown almost all extracellular matrix components and can be found in diseased tissue in the body.

Mucositis is the infection of the mucosa which often happens with a dry mouth or when dentures and other restorations block saliva.

Nasal Dilator allows us to breathe more freely. If you cannot get enough oxygen in through our nostrils our body automatically switches to mouth breathing to provide the required oxygen to the bloodstream, which results in increased snoring, especially if we happen to be sleeping on our back.

Nutcracker effect: to crack a nut one should put it as near the hinge for that is where the greatest pressure can be easily exerted. Occlusal failure or Vertical Loss happens when every tooth loses enamel or restorative material on the top of the tooth and a collapse of the bite occurs.

Occlusal wear: Opposing cusps from chewing teeth hit against fillings wearing them down since enamel or porcelain is harder.

Occlusion: is the bite or contact point between your upper and lower teeth. Grinding can wear away the occlusion.

Onlay fills a hole in the tooth and and covers some of the sides and cusps.

Open margins can allow food collection and bacteria to cause decay under crowns and other restorations.

Operatory is the area where the dentist treats the patient and includes the dental chair, light, and cabinetry.

OSA or Obstructive Sleep Apnea: read what is written on Sleep Apnea Excess tissue in the back of the mouth obstructs airflow causing lack of oxygen.

Osteocytes are cells which initiate healing and shaping of bone after an infection, extraction, or remodeling of bone.

Pericoronitis is an infection of the tissue around an erupting tooth (usually a 3rd molar! It can also be a cause of bad breath in an otherwise healthy person. This often happens to people under heavy stress and lack of sleep such as final exam week.

Periapical Abscess is the result of a dying or dead tooth. The necrotic tissue or bacteria that has invaded the tooth has caused the pulp to die and the tissue in the root or roots to become infected or liquefied. The ligaments at the end of the root is destroyed and fluids or gases fill in the area destroying bone. This is a good sign that you need a root canal.

Periapical X-ray captures the entire crown and root of the tooth.

Periodontal Disease includes simple gingivitis (red or swollen gums), bone recession (the vertical loss of bone, pocket-formation (loss of bone over 4 mm. and through the dura -bone into the spongy bone, and furcation formation (bone loss between roots). Bone can recede at an incline which is called "Ramping," and which tends to trap more food. It is a common disease which forms around = "perio," the tooth = "dontal," affecting the fiber, gum tissue, and bone.

Plaque is sticks to teeth and consists of bacteria, food, saliva and dead cells.

Pocket formation is the main cause of serious periodontal disease. and that is why we probe to measure the depth of the "hole" or defect. It is easy to understand why food and bad bacteria will collect in these pockets causing the pockets to increase in depth or width. We must keep these areas clean or use surgery to eliminate them.

Prebiotics help the good microorganisms (Probiotics) in the gut metabolize nutrients to promote our bodies health. They maintain good metabolic, skin, and organ health, and a healthy immune system by preventing a leaky gut.

Prophy or prophylaxis is a tooth cleaning and one agent in cleaning teeth is the rubber cup.

Pulp is the living tissue inside the tooth which includes blood vessels, nerves, and specialized cells called odontoblasts, fibroblasts, plasma cells and macrophages. It is the soft nerve center and lifeblood of the tooth which is protected by the hard-external enamel and dentin.

Quadrants: your mouth is divided up into four quadrants-2 upper and 2 lower each covering ½ the arch from back molars to front teeth. Receding gums happen as a result of abrasion (toothbrush, acid, abrasive toothpaste or salt) or from forces which push the teeth forward or outward when braces or appliances push teeth, or from grinding of teeth, or from irritations such as from crowns or veneers, or from any other force that causes the tooth to move or rock.

Radiolucency: a dense tissue or object appears whiter on an x-ray. The brighter the radiolucency the denser the material; and very dense is metal.

Resin Cement is a synthetic resin cement used to seal or cement white fillings, crowns and other restorations. The resin cement is stronger than the powder-liquid cements which are still used to cement some crowns and onlays.

Retrognathic: or Class II bite is when the upper teeth are far forward in comparison to the lower teeth- usually a small mandible.

Root Canals: There are 3 types of Root Canals: *One canal* for Anterior teeth *Two canals* for Bicuspids; *Three canals* for Molars. Most Root Canals require a build-up filling and crown since dead teeth are more brittle. However, some DO NOT and that is why you may want a second opinion – Since a Crown and Buildup can be very expensive. In certain situations, a crown can weaken a tooth and not strengthen it. Example: in lower anterior teeth or upper lateral incisors that have thin necks. The root canal requires the removal of any nerve and blood vessels which might still be alive in the roots. The idea is to stop the ~infection in the tooth from spreading and thus stopping the pain and saving the tooth. There is nothing poisonous in a root canal.

Signature Organ is a phrase Dr.Hofmann uses to describe our unique organ that expresses who we are & is the pathway to health: The Mouth

Stroke (ischemic) : impairs part of the brain causing numbness or loss of nerve control permanent or non-permanent. Often the stroke is related to plaque from the jugular arteries, high blood pressure, high stress, and narrowing of arteries in the brain.

Sub-lingual Salivary gland helps deposit calculus (tartar) on your lower front teeth. This gland is often very active when you are stimulated by your senses.

Sub-Mandibular Salivary gland is the primary producer of calcium in saliva.

Super Floss or 3-N-One Floss: has 3 parts including a foam sponge section to carry medication into hard to get areas between teeth and under bridges or around implants. There is a hard tip to thread under bridges and a regular floss area. If you use toothpicks, take care as they can break off in deep areas.

Syncope is the same as fainting. Many factors are related to it including overheating, dehydration, heavy sweating, exhaustion, standing up too quickly, heavy stress, lack of sleep, and fear.

Tetrahydrocannabinol or THC is responsible for most of marijuana's psychological effects. It acts much like the cannabinoid chemicals that our body produces naturally.

TMJ or TMD: Temporal Mandibular Joint or Disorder points to the double joint of the jaw which has cartilaginous disks moving back and forth as you chew. Popping means one or both disks are not moving in sync with the eminence of the condyle. The disk cushions the joint against the Temporal part of the skull. Car accidents and other injuries to the jaw can cause tears into supporting ligaments or perforation of the disk. Pain can happen near the front of the ear where the joint is located. Muscles in the cheek, neck, and back of the head can also become sore. Some people have a jawbone that locks or have pain when chewing or opening wide. Some may have headaches, dizziness, earaches, hearing problems, upper shoulder pain, toothaches, and ringing ears.

Tongue: Physicians know that the tongue is a good barometer to measure levels is a graphic tongue" for instance is due to the deficiency of Vitamin B. The mouth often is the first organ to show the doctor signs of auto- immune disease, some multi-organ syndromes, and other genetic disorders. If you have a sore or pain in your tongue or mouth that does not go away see your dentist immediately.

Veneers are usually made of porcelain or composite materials and cover just the front part of a tooth- usually the front teeth.

Xerostomia is dry mouth resulting from reduced or absent salivary flow.

Xylitol is absorbed more slowly than sugar with a less caloric value and it does not affect blood sugar levels. Chewing Xylitol gum stimulates saliva and can decrease cavity rates and help bone and gums. It is natural to the body and like sorbitol is an alcohol-sugar or polyol.

Zirconia or ceramic crowns are extremely strong, cosmetic in looking and yet non-abrasive. Good for use on Implants.

We have 3 Types of Teeth:

1)   **Incisors** are our front teeth which includes four upper and lower canines and 8 flat incisors - 4 on the upper and 4 on the lower.

2)   **Bicuspids** are located behind the canines, have two cusps, and the mouth typically has 4 of them- often the 1st Bicuspids are extracted for braces which constricts the arch and can create a smaller airway space.

3)   **Molars** are the large, chewing teeth with 4 or more cusps, and often the 3rd molars (or Wisdom Teeth) are extracted because they fail to erupt in proper position. The 1st Molars erupt at the age of 6 and therefore tend to show more wear. Second Molars erupt by the age of twelve and are key to supporting the 1st Molar. The contact between these two teeth is the widest in the mouth and therefore, requires more attention in cleaning with dental floss. We have an upper and a lower arch of teeth, each with sixteen teeth- unless you are born with less! You are better off having your 3rd molars extracted when you are young since the roots are shorter and everything heals quicker.

CHAPTER THIRTEEN
Great Thoughts & Facts
to Smile About

A PERFECT FIT:

By nature, a dentist should be a perfectionist and should be aware of the patient's unique needs. Everybody is unique and different and so are teeth. A cosmetic, white filling on a back molar may last many years in the mouth of a petite woman, but not under the pressures of the muscular male jaw. Aggressive wear can also happen with porcelain crowns or bridges. Realizing everyone is different, there are many other factors that can determine a healthy mouth.

Here are some of those factors: 1) Tooth position and angle; 2) Habits and Diet; 3) DNA and familial influences such as cultural or family habits; and 4) Extraneous influences such as sports, your job, your standard of living, your cleanliness, and past radiation exposure, diseases, and conditions. Simple habits like washing your hands before eating, rinsing with water after a meal, or having two toothbrushes will help control bad bacteria and acids. The following other facts and ideas will help you.

The area where two teeth contact side by side in the mouth is called the interproximal area. This is where most gum disease happens. The main cause is food being trapped between these teeth. Therefore, people use floss to remove it. If you have already lost bone in these areas, you will need to keep these areas extra clean. Methods to use include flossing with super-floss soaked in chlorhexidine or chlorine dioxide; rinsing with a combination of zinc chloride and chlorine dioxide; stopping sugar and junk food habits; and consuming xylitol and healthy foods like raw vegetables. Read Chapters 16 & 23 for more information.

1) After taking an antibiotic for swelling around a tooth, you should rinse with a warm saltwater to help draw the antibiotic to the infection. This will also soften the infection intra-orally and allow drainage of pus. Do not use warm or cold compresses outside of the mouth for it can "harden" or misdirect the infection.

2) If you have just had a temporary crown or *veneer* placed, the dentist may warn you not to floss up and down. The solution is to gently pull the floss out

the side so you will not lift the temporary off.

3) When there is a difficult treatment, the dentist will refer you to a specialist who will advise you and give you treatment options. Implants are a great solution to replace a tooth or many teeth, but they are expensive.

4) There are many foods which help fight tooth decay two of which are dark chocolate and Edam cheese. Whole milk is better for your teeth than skim milk and an apple a-day does help teeth but stay away from apple juice. Xylitol is a *prebiotic*-like food that supports oral and intestinal probiotic bacteria while protecting teeth and bone. Prebiotics help good bacteria while controlling the spread of bad ones. In the colon xylitol forms butyrate which helps support and heal cells of the colon lining. It also helps stop inflammation and infections related to *Candida Albicans* and microbes that can cause leaky gut.

5) When you have pain, record where the pain is coming from and the time of day when it happens. Pain in the morning may point to a different problem and solution than pain at night.

6) Know your own mouth anatomy and where potential problems may arise in the future. Learn the meaning of the acronym CLEARS in Chapter 16. Eat a good balanced diet with a lot of vitamin B and C and remember it matters how you cook your food! Caramelization or over-cooking proteins and carbohydrates can create cancer causing compounds or acrylamides. If you are going to have sugary and/or acidic foods eat them at mealtime only; otherwise the excess sugar can cause tooth decay, periodontal disease and many gut problems.

7) When you snack switch to proteins and non-acidic foods such as cheese, turkey, non-fried chicken, unsweetened yogurt, avocado, salad or salty nuts. Replace regular sugar with xylitol which counters bad bacteria, acids and odors.

8) Studies show that when adding zinc to toothpaste or an oral rinse decreases bacterial growth, plaque and calculus formation, improving taste & mouth odor. Zinc in the diet is important if you are pregnant or elderly. Eat eggs, legumes, seafood, nuts, seeds, and chicken.

9) If you cannot afford dental care call the area's local dental society, dental school, or churches for a dental referral. Many insurance companies such as Aetna and Cigna have discount plans that work very well.

10) A rewarding part of healthcare is being able to help others. There are now many versions of the 3-headed toothbrush which has 3 sets of brushes aimed onto the top and sides of teeth. These can help you clean the teeth of a handicapped or physically compromised loved one. Or you may provide them with a good xylitol chewing gum which will stimulate salivary flow while helping to cleanse food stuck around the teeth and gums. In the process of helping others you will be motivated to keep your own teeth cleaner and your mouth healthier.

11) You might have an inventive idea. One desperate lady came to Dr. Hofmann with a painful unilateral partial denture for a missing lower molar and told him she could not wear it. This type of mini-partial denture tends to irritate the thin edentulous ridge of bone on the lower jaw. He experimented by hollowing out the hard plastic, replacing it with soft pliable silicone reline material. It solved the problem! A good dentist needs to think outside the box for innovation is one of the hallmarks of dentistry.

12) There may soon be answers for your unique problem or syndrome. For instance, the testing of saliva is a new science that will save many lives. It can match your DNA to a specific medication that you can or cannot take and determine what bad bacteria are hiding in your mouth. It can detect what drugs a person is allergic to and help diagnose auto-immune problems that cause bone loss, joint problems or inflammation. Over 27,000 people die each year from allergic reactions to drugs and medications. Uncontrolled inflammation and a bad diet can eventually cause the breakdown of tissues and organs. This includes many subtle problems such as poor night vision, memory loss, and attentiveness. Be willing to break bad habits such as chewing on ice before you break fillings and teeth. A change in lifestyle can save you a lot of money and save your life.

CHAPTER FOURTEEN
From *"WOW"* 2 *"WHOA"*

We are blessed to have established institutions and dental associations that work to protect consumers and patients. This is the "Golden Age" of Dentistry which is more reason for all professionals to focus attention on how to improve the integrity of all components in their various fields of practice. The examples below are just a few solutions related to general dentistry:

Example: 1

A) Patients of different ages and sexes need different treatment plans. Not every patient will bite as hard as the rock-jawed boxer. Those who do have heavy jaw muscles need extra strong restorations. Certain types of bridges, dentures, veneers, fillings, onlays, and crowns may not work. In contrast the petite woman may have a much lower chance of quick recovery from a difficult jaw related surgery. Discuss this with your oral surgeon.

B) Porcelain Crowns on 2nd molars can break easily due to the nutcracker effect of chewing pressure. The 2nd molars are shorter than 1st molars due to the hinge effect and therefore there is often less room for porcelain and metal. This is one good reason why dentists use the full Zirconia crowns which are very strong even when made thin. If you do have a crown with broken porcelain on metal, the tooth is still protected with the metal layer, but you should get it replaced before the upper tooth drifts downward. This is also true for partial dentures. Dr. Hofmann had a recent patient who broke his cast denture clasp. He replaced the broken clasp by shaping a thick round-wire and embedded it in the acrylic; the patient liked it better than the original cast clasp. This type of clasp is more flexible, stronger, and retentive.

Example: 2
A) There is a new product, Silver Diamine Fluoride or SDF which can halt tooth decay quickly and cheaply. It is especially effective for children's teeth and has been shown to stop even deep widespread decay. The bacteria killing micro-particles of silver work layer by layer inside a cavity, killing bacteria and rescuing teeth without pain. Often the patient does not need to be numbed! Placing many layers of potassium iodide over the SDF will help prevent the dark color normally associated with silver oxidation.

A white filling can then be placed over it. This is an excellent solution for anyone with rampant decay or who is incapacitated. Other uses include decay at the neck of teeth, decay under crowns, or decay which has cratered teeth beneath the gum level. Dr. Hofmann has used it to save crowns.

B) It has taken a long time for Silver Diamine Fluoride to be approved by the FDA since the Thalidomide scare decades ago. This product has been used extensively in many parts of the world for the last 5 years with great success. Even though it has saved teeth in thousands of mouths it has only recently been approved for use on adults here in America. Hopefully full approval for children will happen soon.

Example: 3

A) Are you a procrastinating patient who puts off treatment? Have you put off treatment for years and suddenly have an emergency? Like the traveling-through patient, you may require a temporary treatment that is strong enough to last months or until you can see your dentist. Many emergency situations call for root canals or extractions. If you lose a tooth, a quick cosmetic solution is a flipper with an attractive tooth. This is a removable partial which is very reasonable to make and can be done in just hours if the dentist has a good replacement tooth. A great help is the dentist who stocks up on replacement denture teeth for a quick cosmetic fix!

One recent male patient with heavy jaws broke his denture multiple times, so Dr. Hofmann quickly improvised a metal "staple" which reinforced the weak areas. Finding a dentist to do these repairs or fabrications in just hours is becoming difficult. Another very good solution is for the dentist to use the anterior tooth that is extracted as a pontic or bridge to keep the gap filled. By cutting off the root of the extracted tooth the crown part can then be glued to the adjoining teeth on each side with tooth-colored cosmetic composite.

B) When a tooth is removed the most common replacement option offered is an implant. Most people cannot afford them, and some are left in fear putting off treatment. People in desperation should not be taken advantage of. They should be given good options to fit their age, economic level and immediate need without having to wait a long time. Implants are a very good treatment, but many patients cannot afford them. Sinus lifts, bone grafting, and implants with custom abutments are too expensive for many. Every dentist should take courses on how to properly treat the elderly in order to understand their unique needs. Many do not want fancy or expensive care.

Example:4

A) A careful observation by parents and dentists is important in catching sleep disorders quickly. In children it can be as simple as watching how they sleep. Snoring is a definite sign as well as sleeping with their heads back. Parents, if you have any concerns take a video or picture of your sleeping child and share it with your pediatrician! Another sign is a collapsed look in and around their nose, which is called the maxilla and an intruded (retrognathic mandible). Some call this the flat-face look and we should do all we can to counter the collapse of the palatal arch. Expanding the palate with a Bionator, Maxillary Rapid Expander, or the ALF appliance is a great solution. Check these out online. There are orthodontists and general dentists who offer this option.

In adults the signs of sleep disorders are many. It is easy to see how Obstructive Sleep Apnea and Excessive Sleep disorder creates social, family, school, and work problems that have a huge impact on a person's life. Tragically that often leads to depression, car accidents, and suicide. One simple surgery which can help is the release of a tongue tie which is the removal of tissue holding the tongue down into the floor of the mouth. Appliances that reposition the jaw, CPAP and Nasal Dilators can also help and should be considered after a good sleep study. Other possible solutions for adults are a good snore-guard or a lower mouth guard to release and open the bite. Find a physician and dentist who have experience with Sleep Apnea and other disorders.

B)   Both the dentist and the hygienist need to be aware of symptoms related to sleep apnea. A bulky denture can block the airway during the day and it should not be worn at night. A well-designed appliance can move the jaw forward and improve the airway space. The jaw has a double hinge joint and by opening the back part of the bite just 2mm, you can create an opening of 4mm for breathing, as shown in Figure 2. Nasal Dilators which open the nostrils also help the patient breathe more freely.

An Ear, Nose, and Throat specialist should be consulted when it looks like tonsils and adenoids are blocking the airway - which may be why the child is snoring. One good solution is to use appliances which can expand the palate and widen the lower jaw at a young age. Extracting the four bicuspids may create problems by allowing the collapse of the palatal arch and eventually restricting the airway space. The dentist who observes this collapse should spend time talking to parents and their physicians about potential sleep disorders.

Example: 5

A) If you have money problems and have not seen a dentist in a long time, you might ask the dentist if you can have a cleaning done in two appointments. Your teeth may have a lot of stains and buildup of the hard plaque called calculus. The most affected teeth are the lower teeth where saliva pools. Dividing the tooth cleaning into two appointments with two payments will help your budget. Have the most inflamed area treated first. At the next visit the cleaning can be completed, and another evaluation done to see how well the first area is healing. This is also an opportunity for the dentist to measure your oral hygiene skills and reinforce any needs that you may have.

B) There are lecturers who teach dentists how to make more money by breaking up the initial appointment into two separate appointments so they can charge for two exams. Many patients go to an initial visit thinking they are going to have a cleaning done. This does not happen because the dentist tells them they need a deep cleaning first which will cost from $90 to $1200. The $90 or more is charged to them upfront even if they have 100% coverage for preventive treatment. This is because deep cleanings are under basic coverage and not preventive, requiring that you pay 20% plus your $50 to $100 deductible. Usually this deep cleaning involves 2-4 separate visits, each requiring the use of some form of numbing. This is often the way bait-and-switch coupon advertising works. *The patient will end up paying a lot more for what they thought would be a "free cleaning."* Also, if the dentist charges you for two exams, the payment for either the first limited exam or the next new patient exam will not be covered by many insurance companies and you will have to pay.

Example: 6

A) If an old amalgam is dark but the margins are good, leave it alone. If the margin is not leaking but is just corroded, ask the dentist to just polish the margin. When an amalgam is done correctly, they have some of the best margins and are very strong. The amalgam may not look pretty, but Dr. Hofmann has many amalgams in his mouth which have lasted over 40 years. He knows that any substitute will be weaker and will erode more easily, potentially undermining the strength of the tooth. White fillings on back teeth wear away even faster in patients who grind or are heavy chewers. He warns that many of us are living longer and so we need extra strong fillings. Many centenarians living healthy lives have old amalgams which protect the bite and teeth, and allow them to chew well. Removing them would only complicate their health.

"Yes," we should try to find alternatives to amalgam and utilize safe ways to remove them to protect city water, but amalgam is still a good restoration for those who want it. Throughout his career Dr. Hofmann has observed more poorly designed crowns and weak white fillings than poor amalgams. Poorly designed crowns can cause gum disease and destroy opposing teeth, but the holistic community often has no clue. Amalgams help a lot of men chew hard.

B) Many Cosmetic crowns will attract more food and demand more care than a natural tooth with a good white filling or amalgam. Cosmetic crowns on front teeth can cause recession of the gum collar resulting in "ugly" or unattractive root-margins in just months or a few years. This may be a genetic issue or operator failure in design and construction. Typically, a well-placed and polished glass-ionomer type white filling will not cause this kind of recession. The recession may continue even when the crown is replaced. As indicated throughout this book, Dr. Hofmann believes in conservative low-impact dentistry due to these unexpected hazards. If you grind your teeth, a good night guard might prevent the failure of the weaker white fillings.

Example: 7

A) Every effort should be made to protect healthy enamel and core strength of the tooth. The smaller the filling the longer it will last. A conservative dentist will use techniques that preserve enamel and reduce the removal of important enamel structures. The new SDF material will allow us to fill teeth in tough areas since it can kill decay without the drill. Traditionally the best process is removing decay in 3 stages starting with a high-speed drill to open the area for access. A slow speed drill is then used to excavate the decay. Finally, a spoon excavator is used to remove decay layer by layer. This technique conserves the tooth structure and prevents accidental exposure of the nerve. A tooth-colored filling can then be placed. SDF can be used with these steps to insure complete decay removal.

B) Dr. Hofmann started off his career in a building where every doctor smoked. There were two physicians and three dentists. Doctors should set an example and should treat their patients based on how they would want to be treated.

Example:8

A) Geriatric patients often need special attention. Patients and caregivers need to know the importance of keeping the back teeth clean, especially in those who are incapacitated. Bacterial plaques stick onto those back teeth and can possibly be inhaled causing pneumonia. Using a mouth rinse to help control the bacteria is also advised. Some of Dr. Hofmann's favorite patients are the elderly, and many require special attention due to the dry-mouth syndrome.

Over 500 commonly used pharmaceutical drugs or medications cause dry mouth which in turn causes both tooth decay and periodontal disease. Other than decreasing the amounts of those medications there is no easy solution, and therefore, individuals should go to both their dentist and physician for good advice. Under a doctor's care there are medications which can help a dry mouth. There are also many over-the-counter products including special mouth rinses, xylitol toothpastes, xylitol gum and mints, and anti-bacterial xylitol mouth sprays which can help counter bacteria and acids. Symptoms of dry mouth include difficulty speaking, tasting, chewing or swallowing; stickiness or dehydration of the mouth mucosa, cracked lips, a lingering dry or sore throat, and burning sensations. Sjogren's syndrome is a severe form of dry mouth that requires special attention and medications.

B) Special care and attention should be given to the Geriatric Patient. A great example was Dr. Hofmann's 87-year-old mother who lived far away and had an important canine tooth snap at the root. It had supported a 3 Unit-bridge and she was told by a top dentist in her area that she would need an extraction and two implants. She did not want any implants and so she flew up to see Dr. Hofmann who did a root canal and then placed a male-female attachment on the root and for a metal cosmetic partial denture. It was strong, retentive, functional and comfortable. She loved it and wore it until she died 7 years later. It saved her a lot of money, time, grief, and pain. He was so concerned by this lack of appropriate care and treatment planning by that high-powered dentist, that he called up his old dental school and talked to the dean's office. He motivated them to set up a special program emphasizing the needs of geriatric patients.

Example: 9

A) Patients in difficult situations or deep emotional need should be listened to and encouraged. A complex treatment may not be the best. Crowns, bridges and implants require multiple visits. Simple white fillings or a glass-ionomer hybrid filling on top of Silver Diamine Fluoride (SDF) can make a tremendous difference on how a patient with rampant decay looks and feels about themselves. Catching rampant decay early is key to saving teeth and can help people overcome their addictions. Many of these dark black or brown root cavities can be treated with self-adhesive.

tooth-colored. fillings. And now with SDF treatment we can destroy difficult to get decay without a needle or a drill. It can kill bacteria near the nerve or hiding in a deep hole or cavity and under a crown. SDF can work in multi-layered decay killing bacteria layer by layer and has been used for over 8 years in Australia. Although used in many countries, it was only recently allowed into the United States.

B) The selling of expensive crowns, bridges and implants was a topic of many seminars. One seminar promoted the idea of doing a "15-Minute Crown" to save time. The focus was on how dentists can save money by doing quicker work when the real the message should be just the opposite. Crowns should not be done fast. The idea in making a good crown is shaping perfect parallel walls for retention and great margins for gum health. A patient expects a crown to last a long time. A poor crown design or a bad cementing in of the crown can quickly decrease a crown's life and maybe the life of the tooth. A good crown must have tight contacts which will keep food from wedging between the teeth. Chapter 26 will help you learn how to keep the crown clean. Dentists should act honesty and not just SELL-and-SELL!

Example: 10

A) Using appliances which open the maxillary suture line in a child with a small mouth is a very good way to expand or shape the mouth for both the airway and the larger permanent teeth which will be erupting from ages 6-16. This is what is called the science of dental orthopedics and when used in a timely way can save many parents time, money, and worry. It will either decrease the child's time in braces or eliminate the need altogether. Functional appliances can be used to open the bite allowing the jaw to grow forward and out. This helps to stop tooth crowding, excessive over bites, and reduces the requirement for extractions.

B) Missing front teeth in children can be a big challenge for the Orthodontist. Parents may make the mistake of demanding that all gaps be closed. They may not understand the dangers of closing wide gaps due to missing permanent teeth especially if the gap is only on one side of the mouth. Parents must be aware of potential complications in moving teeth across the mid-line of the mouth. Inter-spacing teeth so there are many small gaps can cause future functional and cosmetic problems. Often a child is better off with one wide gap of equal width on each side. This will allow tooth implants to be placed as they grow older. Consult with your Orthodontist and general dentist.

CHAPTER FIFTEEN
<u>Can You Handle the Truth?</u>

<u>FROM BAD TO UGLY</u>: Most people have heard about the massive cases of Medicaid fraud committed by certain doctors around the country. These are rare, but according to the insurance industry, fraud in a smaller scale is much more prevalent. Patients need to be cautious of treatments which seem out of the ordinary and then make the effort to get a second opinion.

If you are being told you need two root canals be suspicious. At times dentistry is practiced by people without a license. In one case a dentist who lost his license in the U.S. moved to Mexico and practiced there. Other cases involve people pretending to be dentists. This is the reason why State Boards require dentists to exhibit their license in a visible area for patients to view. These infractions are the exception and the patient can check online with their State Board of Dentistry. Just type in the name of your state and then "State Board of Dentistry."

Most of the cases involve dentists who were licensed in other countries and moved here. Other forms of illegal dentistry are procedures done by unlicensed hygienists or restorations done by labs without the direct authority of a dentist.

In Dr. Hofmann's small practice, he has seen many patients who were told they needed fillings and expensive restorations which were not necessary. Many were told they needed extensive Deep Cleanings or what is called "Scaling and Root Planning" when the evidence indicated they did not. They came to him for a second opinions with treatment plans in the thousands of dollars. He mentions some of these cases in the book as a warning to you.

One case mentioned earlier, involved a handicapped gentleman who had been having his teeth cleaned and checked at his office for many years. Because he could not drive, he walked over to a dentist just down the street from him and was told he needed thousands of dollars in periodontal surgery and deep cleaning. None of this was necessary. He did not need any treatment! In another case, a Bible teacher and full-time missionary went to a dentist and was told he needed multiple fillings and a series of those deep cleanings. Dr. Hofmann carefully checked every tooth and determined that this surgical treatment plan was baseless. No special treatment was necessary.

Dr. Hofmann's version of the classic Hollywood line is, "You want the truth? Are you sure you can handle it!" What are the institutions that we assign to protect us doing anything about this? Are they doing all they can to warn us? I hope so, but it appears little is being done to drive public discourse. Who is exposing fraud? The media has reported on corporate influence peddling such as gift giving and other rewards to win over doctors to their products and equipment. Recently they exposed faulty medical products not approved by the FDA that were sold overseas to unsuspecting doctors and patients.

Try to digest this: 1) If a patient is told they need $3000 worth of treatment that is baseless and has no merit, then goes to another dentist who agrees with the patient's suspicions, the understanding is no real "malpractice" has happened since the treatment was never consummated. 2) If the patient does not realize the treatment is bogus and goes ahead and has the treatment done, will they ever discover the truth? And if the patient later suspects foul play, where is the clear evidence now that the work has been done? Is there a good solution?

If a patient is wise enough to walk out of the dental office before any treatment is started and then reports it to another dentist who has clear evidence showing those procedures are unnecessary, how should this be reported to authorities? Is it enough to just tell the patient to report it to their insurance company and to the Peer Review of their local dental society? There are cases where gross negligence or faked treatment was discovered by the new dentist who took over on old practice. The evidence was in the charts, x-rays and mouth of the patients.

During his career Dr. Hofmann reported similar cases and had threats made on his practice. A few forms of retaliation used against him were as follows:

1) There is the "lawyer" that comes by the office and verbally threatens you.
2) Or the "patient lawyer" who seeks treatment and then verbally states that something is wrong with your office. They give off-hand suggestions that you should not criticize such and such practice or else a they will file a complaint.
3) And another is the patient who comes in once and makes up a false report to undercut the office on Yelp.

When that dentist makes every effort to contact the "offended" patient there is no response. These retaliations discourage dentists from reporting cases. Unfortunately, many successful scams or deceptive practices occur against those patients without insurance and the poor, since they do not have a third party to validate the treatment.

Another area of potential deception is the tooth with a "craze line" that is magnified with an intra-oral camera to scare the patient into getting a crown made. Minor craze lines are not true cracks, and do not need to be crowned. A major craze line or crack that is sensitive should be repaired. A good treatment is a stainless-steel crown to protect it from fracture until the sensitivity disappears. If there is no sign of swelling or inflammation, consider crowning it. Most simple craze-cracks do not threaten the life of teeth and can easily be repaired if they fracture. A way to protect these teeth is to wear a hard-surface night guard.

Do not be scared by intra-oral camera pictures showing "black spots" on teeth which can be stains that do not require filling. The probe must stick into a hole for it to be considered a true cavity. If you are an adult who has not needed a filling for what seems forever, get a second opinion when you are told you need a series of fillings in these tiny pits.

There are other dental procedures which can compound problems in the mouth such as traditional bridges that do not contact opposing teeth or crowns which have open contacts. An open contact between two back molars as show in Fig. 4, will allow food to collect causing bone loss. It is important that nothing hits too hard or uneven when you close your teeth together. If you feel a high spot when closing or if your teeth do not touch evenly on the right and on the left, make sure you ask the dentist to grind down the spot before you leave.

Dentists take great pride in creating well-contoured lifelike forms when creating restorations. This is very important to the long-term health of the mouth and the patient's well-being. As in medicine, the Hippocratic Oath must be honored. Dentists and hygienists should take every effort to do no harm and do everything possible to help patients.

In conclusion, most dentists are doing a great job protecting your teeth and gums. If a dentist says you need many fillings when you know you do not need any, get a second opinion? If a dentist says you need expensive deep cleanings which you suspect are not necessary see another dentist. And if necessary send a letter to the Texas State Board. This type of deception is not easily adjudicated; after all the treatment has not been performed? How should society hold these dentists accountable? Should we just say, "let the buyer beware," and be done with it? For instance, Dr. Hofmann recently did an exam on a sixteen year-old patient who was told she needed four white fillings. There was no evidence of decay anywhere! At one time he would call those dental offices up to ask why their treatment plan was fabricated.

From Amalgam to the Amazing Xylitol

Some patients have a hard time finding a new dentist after the retirement of their old dentist. Suddenly they are faced with a diagnosis that requires expensive treatment. This is when a new dentist should gently show the patient each problem with clear x-rays and mirror in-hand while a treatment plan is considered. The idea is to win the patient's trust by explaining every step of the diagnosis and treatment. The patient will see the problems and be part of the corrective treatment. If you are a procrastinating patient realize both decay and periodontal disease can form quickly in acid saliva and therefore, learn preventive techniques to neutralize bad bacteria and avoid acids.

Some people are totally against the use of fluoride and amalgam. Good science does not support this. There are hundreds of studies around the world that do not support these contentions. People who have sensitivities or allergies to metals should not have them. They should remove old amalgams, but do it with proper equipment. The great majority of people are not impacted by metals resting in or on their teeth. Just as with vaccines we should not dictate the health of others by our doubt or fear.

Attacks on amalgam fillings, root canals, and fluoride can be side-shows distracting us from real dangers such as periodontal disease, rampant tooth-decay, colon cancer and a poor diet. Sugar consumption after meals can cause chronic or acute inflammation of gum tissue which allows bacteria to hide and populate. They can accumulate enough acid to destroy bone and to mass produce enzymes that can affect the heart, pancreas and other organs. We will discuss more about the dangers of periodontal disease later.

The amalgam alloy placed in your mouth was created by mixing mercury with particles of silver, tin, copper, and zinc in a sealed capsule. The capsule is only opened after the new metal compound called amalgam alloy is completely triturated or mixed. The mix is placed into the tooth and when it hardens it becomes a strong stable metal. Like other metal alloys the amalgam resists wear and can support heavy chewing. Tooth colored fillings are weaker and should only be used for smaller restorative repairs. Most dentists turn to ceramic or gold crowns, inlays and onlays to replace the large amalgams and rarely use amalgam. The problem is these cast restorations are much more expensive.

Ironically both amalgams and fluoride directly or indirectly help to control local bacterial invasion. There are many people on a tight budget who chew with heavy pressure and who choose the strong amalgam over the weaker tooth colored filling. When the amalgam was placed it was a soft malleable metal which was packed tight against the tooth wall and then burnished against all edges to become an ultra-smooth surface! This type of super smooth contact or margin decreases accumulation of food particles, bacterial colonies and calculus. Many dentists would rather have this kind of strong, ultra-smooth surface in their own teeth. There should be an ad saying, "9 out of 10 dentists prefer amalgam in their mouth." An amalgam placed within a groove or pit can last a lifetime, is simple to place and is very reasonable in cost!

Dr. Hofmann often sees elderly patients with smooth amalgam fillings that are in good shape, yet were placed over 50 years earlier. This is not true for cosmetic white fillings small, medium or large on posterior teeth! The bowling-out effect is a common problem as clearly illustrated earlier in Fig.3.

Patients need to know the options and then decide what they want considering cost and long-term results in their unique mouth. Some patients who chew too hard want amalgams because insurance pays 80% of the fee verses 50% for a $700 to $1,100 onlay or crown. Insurance companies know amalgams protect teeth and are very cost efficient! They know moderate sized amalgams have held up for decades which is much better than white fillings and even many crowns. The insurance standard for the longevity of a crown is only 5-7 years! Many large amalgams are doing well even after 20 to 40 years!

Check out the chapter on "Myths" for more information. A high-end dentist might argue, "Why waste time preserving amalgam fillings when a crown covers the entire tooth." The challenging retort is: "Are you willing to lower your 1000% profit margin and decrease by 50% the charge on those crowns?" Crowns are a major profit center for dental practices and so they promote the removal of amalgams. Many poorly made crowns can attract bacteria, cause inflammation and require extra effort to keep the tooth, gums and bone healthy.

Dr. Hofmann believes whole-body concepts in nutrition are key. Bad bacteria in our sinuses and throat are promoted by sugar. One of these is *Strep mutans* which causes strep throat. Strep floats in our saliva and is part of our normal biofilm. When you are stressed or oral care is weak, they can easily multiply, causing inflammation as they mass-produce acids.

Mouth rinses or toothpaste with essential oils such as eucalyptus oil, Tea tree oil and peppermint oil can help to prevent their spread. The best solution is xylitol in any form placed in the mouth. It can stop *Strep mutans* and stimulate the production of more saliva which helps to wash away them away.

This is a much better solution than taking antibiotics which Dr. Hofmann had to do year-in and year-out for many years. If he did not take penicillin, his dry cough and irritated throat would turn into a serious Strep throat.

Another interesting observation proven by Finnish research is that babies born of pregnant mothers who had taken xylitol were protected up to age of 5. Here is a sugar that can protect us from birth till death. It is such an amazing sugar that the FDA allows it to be classified as "Sugar-Free."

It may surprise you to know that a very effective nasal solution that counters chronic sinusitis or congestion is xylitol in saline solution mixed with some basic essential oils such as oregano oil, eucalyptus oil and tea tree oil. One danger of using too many antibiotics is that it can breed a more resistant strain which will attack us in a stronger way when our immunity is low. Xylitol, however, works in a direct and natural way as it counters many bad microbes including *Candida Albicans*. The bad microbes consume it and can no longer produce acids, inflame tissue or multiply.

Some people have sensitivities to flavorings or additives, especially to cinnamon in toothpaste. If you've developed irritated and chapped lips or a rash around your mouth, and you think your toothpaste is to blame, the first thing to do is stop using it. You can try switching to a brand without any flavoring or other additives and see if your symptoms resolve. Try one with zinc phosphate or xylitol with baking soda or with one or more essential oils.

The number one priority should be the welfare of the patient. This includes cost and diagnostic honesty. The dentist should forewarn the patient of any risks and extra costs due to possible failure. This was exemplified by two people who visited Dr. Hofmann's office as emergency consults. Both had all their amalgam fillings removed and replaced with pre-cured resin onlays and inlays. X-rays showed that almost every restoration was failing with extensive decay underneath and around the margins. The treatment would require multiple extractions, root canals, replacement teeth and implants. Both patients returned to their homelands and so no follow-up was able to be made.

We need honest dentistry and instead of wholesale replacement of amalgams, we should find ways to prevent tooth decay and periodontal disease. Dr. Hofmann has seen patients who were told they needed many expensive and unnecessary crowns. This is a blight on the profession of dentistry. Recently he saw a patient with a decayed and broken front tooth that was told a week earlier that she needed a root canal and crown, yet she was not in pain and her x-ray did not indicate that she needed one. That office told her that it would cost $3000 up front with financing. This was an emotional situation for her since she did not have the money. She had the courage to walk out and ask a friend for advice. Dr. Hofmann was able to save the tooth without a root canal and crown. The treatment he chose saved her a lot of money and was also more cosmetic.

Other patients have surprisingly good situations which are great teaching tools. One frantic patient was having intense stress, eating sweet foods and not flossing. She had not seen a dentist in two years. Dr. Hofmann feared what he might see. He was astounded that she had absolutely nothing wrong. Her mouth was perfect. There was no sign of plaque nor calculus and her gums were immaculate. He did not have to clean her teeth. But he did show her the benefits of a super-soft toothbrush. He encouraged her and asked important questions to learn about her habits, preventive techniques, and diet history. She had a very good perspective on life and seemed very content. He did not try to sell her an ultrasonic toothbrush or mouth rinse.

She is an example of how difficult it is to measure stress and calculus formation. Does a good attitude and heartfelt kindness overcome the effects of stress and anxiety? Do love and faith help? These are difficult questions for the researcher. Are there other factors like exercise or good DNA or a special diet that help create a healthy sustained saliva so that flossing is not necessary? Dentists and patients should take note when less calculus is apparent or when that perfect saliva or mouth is discovered. More data may help us understand why flossing and going to the dentist every six months may not be the complete answer to a healthy mouth. In that person's case flossing and seeing a dentist on a regular basis obviously had nothing to do with keeping her mouth in great condition. We need more evidence-based, bottom-up research and less research based on the profit motive and the desires of special interest groups like the sugar cartel. Understanding how to maintain a very healthy saliva and the science of calculus formation are key to helping us improve the prevention of periodontal disease and thus many other problems.

CHAPTER SIXTEEN
The CLEARS Way to Good Health

What a joy it is to have a clean mouth that CLEARS out disease. Enjoy the optimal feel and the self-cleansing ability of a healthy mouth. To help you remember a way to attain and preserve optimal saliva and tooth health is to use the word "CLEARS" as an acrostic:

1) We want to CHEW slowly so the orally produced enzyme Amylase will do its job and dissolve the sticky starches. When you swallow a bolus of food, it should be partially digested. This acrostic will also remind you to CHEW xylitol gum or mints having 5 to 15 grams a day to CATCH and deactivate acids and bad bacteria. Start with 4-5 grams then work up to 15.

2) We want to drink water or nutritious lite LIQUIDS that have little or no sugar or acids. Stay away from all carbonated drinks and acidic energy drinks while remembering to keep hydrated. This will protect your saliva and teeth.

3) Next, we want to Eat ENRICHING foods and not empty calories. Eat raw vegetables and stay away from processed carbohydrates like potato chips, white bread, snack crackers, cookies, and cake. And remember it matters how you cook food; high heat denatures proteins and sugars creating *carcinogenic molecules.*

4) We can finish off our restaurant meal with a RINSE of the water at your meal table, or at home with your favorite mouth rinse. If water flush it around your teeth and swallow. You can use chlorine dioxide which counters acids or find an over-the-counter rinse such as Listerine with essential oils or zinc chloride to help neutralize bad bacteria and odors. Listerine has a brand new therapy rinse called Listerine Gum Therapy. If you have periodontal disease, you can use these rinses in conjunction with other professional rinses such as stannous fluoride. For more effect do not rinse with water afterwards, instead use super-floss soaked in chlorhexidine to clean any inflamed hard-to-get areas. If you have erosion or a lot of food traps buy a super-soft toothbrush that can get around all curves and corners without hurting fragile tissues. Activated chlorine dioxide will kill both bacteria and spores, and will also neutralize acids which collect in and around the gum collar surrounding teeth.

Here again is the acrostic to remember:

C = Chew slow & digest food using the enzymes in your saliva to help digest them.

L = Learn to Like Liquids with less sugar and more water & say no to lite soft drinks. Use xylitol in your coffee, tea, and/or chew xylitol gum or a mint.

E = Eat Enriching foods with a lot of fiber, minerals, vitamins and proteins.

A = AND

R = Rinse Right before bed with a combination of rinses (chlorine dioxide + a fluoridated rinse or a rinse with zinc chloride) which is especially good for those with mouth odor. Rinse after eating with the drinking water at your table, and then just swallow the water. This will help CLEAR your mouth of food, acids, and bacteria. The last step is to add an "S" to this acrostic for "STOP STRESSING" as you brush and throughout the day:

S = Stop Stressing your teeth by over-brushing and if you have erosion use a super-soft toothbrush in the area. Bad thinking can cause us to brush with heavy stress or to neglect oral hygiene altogether. Close your teeth together as you gently brush in the far back molars where many people fail to brush. By stretching your cheek, you can brush behind the last tooth. Next brush behind your lower front teeth with the brush handle pointed straight up and the bristles perpendicular to the bite. As you brush the area near the neck of the teeth go up and down with bristles angled at a 45-degree angle to the surface.

Buy a set of 4 super-soft toothbrushes at H-Mart and use two per day so each can dry out as you rotate them. This will kill the bacteria and prevent re-contamination. The Korean made super soft brushes are stronger and clean better than any other super soft brush that Dr. Hofmann has seen or used.

As stated in Chapter 8, stress can lead to the grinding of teeth and increase the acidic level of your saliva. Along with acids consumed and acids produced by bad bacteria the acidity of saliva can reach the point of causing the decalcification of teeth. Arginine an amino acid found in many foods, can help to produce a less acidic saliva. It is found in dark green vegetables, nuts, meats, and beans.

Many dentists believe the acidic level of saliva is a factor in the formation of the calculus which can cause serious periodontal disease. It is possible the battery-effect of acids plus electromagnetic currents in the body play a part. The mouth pools saliva filled with positive calcium ions which are attracted to the negative polarity of teeth. The sticky plaque is then hardened by those calcium ions leaving a rock-hard surface which cannot be flossed or brushed off. These rock-like adhesions are made of calcium carbonate and are called "calculus." Bacteria clings to them and if they are not removed gingivitis can become a bone-destroying *periodontitis*. This destructive process will destroy good bone around the roots of teeth. What would you think or do if this kind of bone loss was happening anywhere else in your body? You would probably freak out! And research shows replacing regular sugar with xylitol sugar can help lower the rate of this bone loss.

The battle in your mouth is extremely important. Both hard and soft bacteria laden particles can be inhaled as particle aerosols potentially causing serious and sometimes deadly pneumonia in a weakened individual. Therefore, you do not want bacterial plaque to build up. Anytime bad acid-producing bacteria can cling to a surface in the mouth for a long enough period it will cause either inflammation of the gums or decalcification of enamel or dentin. The challenge is to keep them off those surfaces and allow them to be washed away by rinses, toothpaste, water, or normal mouth function. The best weapon is good saliva. And a great tool to increase the flow of saliva is the use of xylitol. Xylitol will also lower the acidity of saliva, hinder the activity and reproduction of bad bacteria, and help prevent both calculus formation and periodontal disease.

Flossing and brushing the right way is key to the removal of food and bacteria in the hard to get areas between the teeth. If you only floss through the contact without going up and down the walls on each side, pulling and pushing the floss along the curves and dropping down under the collar, then your flossing is less effective. Complicating the access to these areas are pockets in the bone, shoulders and gaps in crowns and fillings and dips and crevices where the roots of teeth bifurcate (the furcation). and other food traps require special attention.

A super-soft toothbrush will allow the unbent bristles to penetrate deep between teeth where bone loss has opened gaps. The bristles in contact with the immediate tooth surface will bend harmlessly. Another excellent solution is to saturate the foamy part of Super-Floss or "3-n-One" dental floss with liquid chlorhexidine or activated chlorine dioxide and use it to floss between teeth. An illustration of this product and how to use the foamy floss is shown on the next page.

HOW TO USE SUPER-FLOSS to PROTECT DISEASED BONY POCKETS:

Use the regular floss section of super-floss to get between the teeth and then use the foamy part like a piece of cloth polishing a shoe. Go back-and-forth pushing it against the far side and then pull forward towards each tooth wall and clean it. This process will leave behind the anti-bacterial agent that soaked the spongy area.

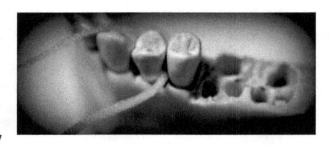

Fig 7

This illustration shows pockets in the bone. The dura-hard bone is the shiny bone, but the spongy bone is the pitted bone near the root sockets. These are pockets where bacteria collect destroying bone. Therefore, we want to get into these areas between the teeth and disinfect them with chemical agents that will kill deep anaerobic bacteria. In the photo the foamy part of the super flood is shown between the teeth. When you pull or push back on it the chemicals will be released. Fluoride can be used to help strengthen the decalcified area with a strong fluorapatite matrix.

Keeping your toothbrush clean and dry is important. A simple way to clean your toothbrush is with soap and water? It is not a good idea to let bacteria grow on your brush and that is why a moist environment is bad. So, keep your brush upright and away from the toilet area. If necessary, you can clean it with hand soap or chlorhexidine. Do not use a cap on the brush head as it can cultivate the common yet virulent Pseudomonas bacteria. Having a second dry toothbrush available is also a good idea since a moist toothbrush can grow bacteria. Dentures and night guards can be kept clean in a homemade solution of a cup of water with a ½ teaspoon of dishwater soap, bleach and white vinegar. Keep your pets away from dentures or they will chew them up!

Getting a new toothbrush when the bristles appear frayed, bent, or discolored is important. There are many toothbrushes to choose from including those with long curved necks and small heads, making them easier to reach behind the last molar and down behind your lower front teeth. Those are two areas where calculus can form without detection causing bone loss. The back molars have wider contacts and therefore act as food-traps, making it important to floss and to brush well on both inside and outside.

For patients with delicate areas such as deep receding gum tissue, Dr.

Hofmann recommends special extra soft toothbrushes made in South Korea labeled either Gold or Silver "Well Being." The thin tipped bristles help get into the sensitive collar and crevices around each tooth without irritating any tender gingiva or eroded root areas. The South Koreans mastered the concept of making an effective and tough super-soft bristle.

Most brands that Dr. Hofmann has seen make the mistake of placing their bristles in tufts that distort and bend over as a group. They then accumulate bacteria. They also do not clean well since individual bristles do not separate and penetrate the curves and delicate collar of the gingiva. If you know of any good super-soft brands, let Dr. Hofmann know at his website: DentistryXposed.com. He wants to keep everyone informed of new information, developments and products. Also leave comments and share any experiences that you have had that are note-worthy. It is also important to note that when a toothbrush manufacturer bundles 8 or more "soft bristles" into a pointed tuft, that tuft becomes much stiffer and can harm delicate tissue or wear away the root surfaces. This is the classic problem with American toothbrushes. Just making the switch to a Korean-type super soft toothbrush can make a huge difference.

Keep in mind that good preventive care begins with what you put in your mouth. Eating healthy food and drink protects every cell, and the nutrients will sustain every organ including the mouth and saliva. If you are behind in your quality care and nutrition, all hope is not lost. Amazing changes can happen in our bodies when we stop bad habits like smoking and stop consuming so much sugar, empty carbs, and fat. In many ways it is like watering, fertilizing and weeding a badly dried out lawn. It can be recovered, but it is going to take tender care and time. And it will be much easier to keep that beautiful thick grass fed and groomed. Prevention is much safer, cheaper, and kinder to the body, soul and mind than having to take medications or treat disease. America has become adept at treating disease and manufacturing drugs. We should adopt better prevention concepts and techniques in order to stop disease trends that are harming millions. These trends include chronic brain and auto-immune diseases, diabetes, cancers, and degenerative joint and vascular diseases - many of which are caused by disease conditions in the mouth and gut.

CHAPTER SEVENTEEN
Scams and Deceptions

"You want to be able to trust your dentist, for the same reason you want to trust your car mechanic: most of us don't have the expertise to evaluate the diagnosis," states Marilyn Bowden from the Article under: "Insurance Scams" June 9, 2017 on the Online page of Bankrate. This may say something about what insurance companies or those who write for them think about the integrity within the field of dentistry. Dr. Hofmann is not in agreement with her comparing dentists to auto mechanics. He believes a great majority of dentists are honest and determined to provide fair treatment for their patients. However, there are many scams in dentistry that he wants you to be aware of.

Marilyn, then quotes James Quiggle, of the Coalition Against Insurance Fraud, who says "While most dentists are ethical it's smart to remember the degree on the wall isn't a guarantee of honesty. Dental scams sink their teeth into unsuspecting patients every year." He continues, "The most frequent dental scams are inflating claims, delivering worthless treatment that patients don't need and billing insurers for phantom treatment the dentist never delivered. Added up, these cons can mean big dollars for a dentist's bank account."

What is not stated in this article is that often these scams are perpetrated on people who do not have insurance. The scammer wants to avoid the extra scrutiny and expertise insurance companies provide in detecting fraud. Marilyn states, "The National Health Care Anti-Fraud Association estimates Americans lose about $68 million dollars each year to health care fraud." These are recent estimates from insurance companies, and do not include the billions potentially scammed over the many decades by payments outside of the insurance industry. Below is a list of scams Marilyn noted in her article:

SCAMS or DECEPTIONS:

1) She quotes, "Phoney-baloney insurance billing: Less-than-honest dental practices may bill insurance providers for more expensive procedures than those actually performed; or fabricate charges entirely." Deep Cleanings versus Regular Cleanings, are a big part of these overcharges and fraud. Those over-charges vary from $70-$250 when a PPO type insurance is used, but total much more with regular insurance or without insurance.

Quiggle continues, "Check your explanation of benefits closely to make sure the bill reflects what procedures the dentist performed."

2) "Submitting multiple claims: Another way, dentists might exaggerate a claim.. to break down a comprehensive procedure such as a root canal into its component parts and charge for each one, even though a single code could be used for the whole procedure." Another example is to charge for the cementing of a crown which should be included in the original price of making the crown. Insurance companies normally catch these infractions.

3) Some procedures are unsupported by scientific evidence and should be avoided," says Dr. Barrett M.D. "In the quackery line," he says, "the clear winner is removal of amalgams." There is a lot of money made in replacement fillings and placement of crowns, inlays, onlays, and bridges.

The promotion of amalgam removal has become a national money maker since restorative replacement is often not necessary. One speaker even claimed 95% of amalgam fillings have decay underneath and should be removed. This claim and others are not supported by research nor by the American Dental Association. In fact, there is more chance for problems around white fillings and crowns than around amalgams! Using only white fillings as replacement restorations is risky as they have a high rate of wear and will allow vertical collapse of the entire bite as shown in figures 2 & 3.

The fact is the FDA considers amalgam fillings safe but there is potential risk from removing dental amalgam. The removal can release metals into the city's water supply. Cities are demanding that dentists install modern amalgam traps on their dental units. High speed suction units in every dental office do a very good job in sucking the particles away quickly before the patient swallows.

Marilyn, goes on to say, "Be skeptical if a dentist recommends implants or bridge work where a simple removable appliance would do." The following should be carefully explained to the patient: 1) Both the cost and risk versus benefits should be carefully explained. 2) Long term consequences of both removal or placement and any special care required to keep it clean. 3) All options that are available including removable partial dentures should be explained. Partials have a big advantage in that they can be removed so that the whole area can be cleaned easily. Although a good clinician can create a very cosmetic and well-shaped restoration many crowns fail at the margin or at contact points resulting in a poor appearance and the collection of food.

Bridges require special cleaning under the pontic that connects the two crowns. Bridges made of porcelain can be too abrasive against lower teeth. A better solution might be an implant or that cosmetic partial denture which is cheaper and can replace multiple teeth in strong acrylic.

The popular porcelain crowns can also cause abrasive destruction on the occlusion of opposing teeth. This was very evident in a case where porcelain crowns had been placed in a staggered formation on upper and lower arches so that no crown hit on another. This checker-board design generated extensive wear on all the natural tooth surfaces. The overall effect was collapse of the entire bite. This is what we call the loss of vertical and the result can be the need for a full mouth rebuild.

Crowns in themselves are not bad. However, the improper use, placement, or design can be disastrous.

Crowns can weaken the intrinsic strength of narrow necked teeth and unsupported root canaled teeth! Dr. Hofmann cautions, "The patient should be allowed to decide, especially in the case of the elderly! Many of these root canaled teeth do not need to be crowned." As stated earlier the top dentist in his graduating class tried to sell my 87-year old mother two implants that she did not need nor want when she broke a tooth on her front bridge.

A male-to-female or ball-and-socket attachment connecting a metal partial to the stable root can work better. This was strong and very esthetic with a total cost of about $1200 – $2000, verses a minimal cost of $9000 to $15,000 for bone grafting, two implants, extraction, and three cosmetic crowns." Dr. Hofmann was so alarmed by the poor treatment plan given to his mother that he contacted the dental school where she lived. He was told that the school would initiate a Geriatric Program to further educate the student dentists on the need to offer a balanced and practical treatment concept for the elderly.

These next three scams are not on Marilyn's list:

1) The Classic "Bait and Switch" Scam: This is often a COUPON SCAM which draws patients to a "cheap offer" of either free x-rays, free Cleaning, free Exam, or a combination discount. This scam usually attracts patients without insurance. The patient is then sold a package treatment involving a series of deep tooth cleanings called Scaling and Root Planning. The patient ends up NOT getting the simple cleaning that they expected. Instead this dental office refuses to do a regular cleaning

or treatment unless a deep cleaning is done first!

This kind of demand was made to Dr. Hofmann when he went in for a simple cleaning and exam. On their New Patient form he indicated that he was an "author," simply because he did not want special attention. The following is his account: "The dentist enlarged my x-rays on a computer screen and then proceeded to explain that I had deep pockets behind the last molars. The problem is those were not periodontal pockets as defined by the science of Periodontics. He then stated that a deep cleaning had to be performed before any regular cleaning could be done! My desire to get a regular cleaning would not be possible in this office, until I paid for the much more expensive deep cleaning. Those so called 'deep pockets' WERE FALSE POCKETS NOT REQUIRING ANY SPECIAL TREATMENT except for a regular cleaning. Probing on the backside of upper and lower 2nd molars will usually show "false pockets" since this is where we naturally have a thick pad of fibrous tissue. This office was trying to convince me that I had periodontal disease and that I would need 4 quadrants of deep cleaning."

This dentist purposefully tried to misinform Dr. Hofmann by showing him areas where the tissue is normally thick and fibrous. A normal cleaning at this PPO office would have cost $75, but a set of 4 quadrants of deep cleanings would have cost as much as $600 without insurance. Multiple this by an average of two patients a day and the profit can easily run over $10,000 per month. If the patient does not have insurance and is not protected by insurance fee schedules, the charges can easily triple. Unfortunately, the incentive to cheat is big and growing bigger since most patients have little idea what is going on. This is an important warning for all who are told that they need expensive deep cleanings.

2) Over the last 43 years, Dr. Hofmann has seen dozens of treatment plans from patients wanting a second opinion from his office, this included many expensive "deep cleaning" treatments that were not necessary. Since Dr. Hofmann prevented these treatments from being performed, they were not reported to authorities. He did advise the patient, to contact the dentist involved and if necessary, to notify the local dental society or the State Board of Dentistry.

Many General Practice dentists and Periodontists can charge as much as $900 to $2000 for a full mouth of deep cleanings. These deep cleanings often include chemical inserts that easily fall out and do little to protect defects. Most deep cleanings are necessary and most dentists are honest. Insurance companies do a good job of monitoring what is necessary and what is fraudulent.

However, patients without insurance do not have protection and do not know what is happening.

As a patient you should seek a second opinion whenever you have any doubt, and demand a copy of the x-rays, especially if you have never had any periodontal issues. This is your evidence! Hopefully this problem is not endemic in countries throughout the world. It is now a requirement that dental offices post the address of the State Board in the reception area for all patients to see. Are you aware of this? Many large cities also have dental societies to help mediate complaints.

3)   This next deception can be a very lucrative one because it falls into a category outside the codes of some insurance companies and the HMO's. This was true 8 years ago, and today it may have less impact since partial coverage under a new code should pay a part of the cost.

This situation is one which motivated Dr. Hofmann to write a letter to state officials. A retired city official came into his office wanting him to extract a tooth. Dr. Hofmann told him his office no longer belonged to his managed care. The patient said he did not trust his designated dentist and that he would pay for the extraction. Looking him in the eye, Dr. Hofmann stated, "This tooth is so loose it moves when you breathe and no one in your Managed Care Program can charge you more than a few dollars under your contract." He agreed to go back to his assigned managed care provider.

Later he returned to Dr.Hofmann's office and showed his receipt for the extraction. Dr. Hofmann could not believe his eyes! It was over a hundred dollars! The bill stated he had also been charged for the placement of a synthetic bone graft! This office was able to make a large profit by using a code which was not restricted by the contracted fee limitation! This was a flagrant abuse of treatment protocol and professional care. There wasn't a bone socket for the graft insert to be placed. This was an ugly example of fraud.

Bone inserts and grafting in general should be carefully evaluated as to the long-term viability of the procedure. We should not be content with just a 5-year prognosis. Bone augmentation or grafting should last for a very long time. This is a good reason to use proven techniques such as the guided tissue regeneration procedure to grow your own bone in a bony defect.

The following are situations or procedures that do not fit the definition of a scam, but are worth listing because they are common and cost the patient a lot:

1) If you have an emergency, help the dentist investigate all the possible causes and location of your pain. One recent Christmas Dr. Hofmann had a series of 6 patients with intermittent pain on one or more teeth. Many of them had been told they would need a root canal. In each case, he discovered either the pain was not related to the suspected tooth or the discomfort could be resolved without a root canal. One had a crown with cusps which were so steep they were hitting at a bad angle. Back teeth should hit straight up and down and not on the slopes. Some of these patients were grinding their teeth due to holiday stress or were chewing too fast on harder foods such as peanut brittle. This caused a strain and pain to ligaments on the tooth and bone.

Doing minor adjustment on the top surface of the tooth can solve the problem. When a tooth is strained it's like a twisted ankle. The ankle with fluids in tissue layers. Likewise, the tooth with its strained ligaments rises upward in the bone socket that holds it in. The space where the tooth attaches to the bone fills with fluids. If this swelling causes the tooth to rise a small amount the tooth will now hit harder against the opposing tooth. Any chewing will cause the tooth to hit harder and harder as it hits again and again resulting in more and more swelling. This vicious cycle can eventually result in the death of the tooth. Therefore, it is very important to seek treatment quickly.

2) Many fillings are done with the pretext that decay has been detected by the dentist's sharp probe. If the probe does not stick into a hole, there is usually no decay penetrating the enamel deep enough to necessitate a filling. Ask your dentist to show you with a mirror how the probe sticks. Shallow defects can be healed with good saliva and remineralization. At times a groove can have an unusual configuration which can hide decay even though the probe does not stick. Also note that a dark stain does not preclude tooth decay and if someone suddenly says you have decay get a second opinion.

3) Night guards are easy to make, and so is it fair to charge 10 to 15 times the expense it takes to make them? The comfortable heat-sunk ortho-plastic night guard can easily be offered at about $200? This helps to motivate the patient to buy and use them. Night guards are especially helpful to protect weak or partially loose teeth in the mouth of a grinder. A dentist can make two of these for the price of one made in a laboratory. The lab designed night guard is thicker, more expensive, often less comfortable, and less likely to be used. However, they can function very well as a lower guard to open the bite wider for sleep improvement or as a TMD treatment appliance. The thicker guard allows the dentist to open and reposition the jaw to protect the joint. There are also specialty appliances which will reposition

the jaw and keep it open in that position during sleep. Some of these are snore-guards. guards. Check with your dentist about other available devices for sleep apnea.

4)   Free Whitening kits are sometimes used to draw new patients to offices. Have you discovered that some of these are worthless and do not work beyond a few weeks? If they are made with a thermoplastic material, they will warp easily due to heat from the body and air. It will then fail to seal the carbamide peroxide whitening agent against the tooth and will allow saliva to neutralize the chemical.   This warping also permits the chemical to escape into the mouth! Excessive use of peroxides can interfere with the calcifying of the enamel and can be an irritation to the mucosa, gums and throat.

A good bleaching tray is made by heat-sinking the soft plastic tight against an accurate stone model impression of your real teeth. This offers a accuracy which will not distort easily, and keeps the solution pressed and sealed against the tooth. It is like a drop of water pressed between two pieces of glass. The patient can then control how many times a day they want to whiten their teeth. They will have full control of the process and if there is sensitivity, they can stop treatment.

Dr. Hofmann enjoyed making these very accurate soft trays with a peripheral seal. They were designed to prevent leakage and protect the gum tissue. People need to understand that fast whitening with heat can shock and cause pain to both teeth and tissue especially in younger people and people with sensitive skin. There seems to be a correlation between sensitivity of the skin with sensitivity of the gum tissue. And as stated earlier, whitening does remove the protective film layer and may over time harm the thin gum attachment at the neck of the tooth.

CHAPTER EIGHTEEN
<u>Opioids, Vaping & E-Cig Crisis</u>

Drug abuse in America has become an epidemic crisis leaving behind a trail of bad teeth, oral destruction, broken families, and death. More people die from drug overdoses than from car accidents. The characteristic "Meth mouth" has blackened, rotting, or crumbling teeth. This tooth decay is caused by the following factors: physiologic changes resulting in dry mouth; the heavy use of sugar products; and the patient's failure to perform oral hygiene. Methamphetamine, otherwise called crystal, ice, glass, and speed is very acidic and will destroy more than just teeth. The tissue destruction is very dramatic.

Statistics show that America consumes 80% of the world's opioids! The Surgeon General's spotlight on opioids warns that over 115 people die per day as a result. The rate of increase was six times higher in 2018 than 1999 and keeps growing. Overdosing is the fourth leading cause of death in America. One small town in West Virginia, with less than thirty-five hundred residents, and two pharmacies prescribed 20.8 million pain prescriptions for painkillers in just ten years. Corporate drug makers promoted these pills to physicians and dentists who then wrote large scripts for patients who claimed to be in pain. As a result, opioids have become the number one prescription drug in America.

It is up to doctors and pharmacies to limit the over distribution of opioids. Opioids left unused are often stolen by others and abused or sold on the market. It's wise for all users to keep them hidden or destroy them when not used. In the 1990's, dentists were the top writers of scrips for Hydrocodone type opioids! There are many ways to reduce use of opioids and one is limiting the prescriptions to an amount that will last only seven days. Some research shows that opioid use has fallen in regions where medical marijuana has been accepted. Medical marijuana may have help to reduce the dependency on opioids.

Related to all of this is the huge casualty rate of the drug wars. From the Congressional research service and other reports, we know that: 1) Of the 237,580 people murdered in Mexico since Jan. 1, 2007, about 44 % were killed in drug cartel-related violence; 2) In the 1st six months of 2019, seventeen thousand were slaughtered; 3) And in the United States an estimated 11.4 million individuals (4.2%) used heroin, misused prescription pain relievers, or did both in 2017. The cartels make over $29 billion a year selling drugs here.

The biggest "cartels," however may be Chinese enterprises! Europe, Japan, Israel, and the U.S. at one time produced 90% of the world's legal drug supplies. China is now the largest supplier. The U.S. has stopped producing both penicillin and aspirin. China has driven the factories in the U.S. out of business. China makes all the crucial Heparin we use to prevent blood clots during surgery. Not too long ago we discovered they sent us defective batches.

On the darker side, China is the biggest producer of compounds for making meth, fentanyl, and other synthetic drugs coming across the border and through our ports of entry. Fentanyl is cheaper and 50 times more potent than heroin. In just six years deaths from fentanyl have increased 1000%. This may be due to criminal elements connected to the Communist party. Why have we not prevented this and why do we allow the spread of Chinese branch banks all over the country that help this black market? Drug abusers are also victims. One problem may be linked to the cargo container trade and the ease of hiding powders. We are paying a very heavy cost for our trade and interchange with China. Will it be possible for us to change our dependency on goods from China? We need to become a nation that practices good eating habits and preventive counter measures.

A big problem in dentistry is that pain in the mouth can be disguised and the average dentists can fall for the lies and deceit. The abuser will often have one or more teeth that are either fractured, decayed or root canaled. He or she will claim the tooth hurts all the time. Yet, they will refuse treatment on that tooth since they want to use it as a future ploy to get more drugs. This is one way to identify the abuser along with the fact they rarely show up for treatment.

The dentist should show compassion to those in pain and to the drug abuser. The best solution is to treat the problem and to then prescribe Tylenol with codeine or ibuprofen. Drugs deplete both the natural serotonin and dopamine levels and so It takes a lot of love and dedicated time to restore the body, mind, and soul. Medical studies show positive emotional support and prayer can go a long way to changing a drug habit. An early mistake Dr. Hofmann made in his career was taking a job with a dentist he did not know. He was hired to help-out a dentist who the manager said was "temporarily sick". Dr. Hofmann was told it would be a short-term job. Later, he discovered the dentist was under investigation by State officials for Demerol abuse. The State Board asked Dr. Hofmann to shutter the practice by finishing up all necessary treatment.

Earlier in this book a replacement for opioids was suggested. This was a synergistic combination of either, ibuprofen or Naproxen taken with a 325 mg.

102

Tylenol or acetaminophen. It is important to note any *NSAID* like ibuprofen can be dangerous if over consumed. Common bad effects can include peptic ulcers, a dry mouth, ulcer disease, acute kidney injury, increased blood pressure, and increased incidence of myocardial infarction (heart attack. The risk of injury is increased in the elderly as well as anyone taking angiotensin-converting enzyme inhibitors, beta blockers (used to control heart rhythm), and certain blood pressure medicines. It is not good for patients who are taking anti-coagulants and immuno-suppressive drugs used to protect implanted organs. People with hypertension and other blood pressure issues should also be very careful.

If you have any of those conditions be sure and consult with your physician or specialist before beginning a course of Tylenol or ibuprofen.

We must work together to defeat America's worst epidemic. Patients should avoid the overuse of any opioid and doctors should do everything possible to lessen pain. The temporary benefits of opioids may be good considering sleep and pain needs. The use of marijuana for medical and recreational use is growing fast, despite studies that show decreased ability to think (cognitive loss in the developing teen and young adult brain. Although cannabinoids in marijuana have beneficial effects cannabis smoke dries out the mouth and contains many of the same toxic compounds found in tobacco smoke including carcinogenic aromatic hydrocarbons. And it has been shown that marijuana is a gateway drug which may lead to chemically addictive drugs. The long-term effects are not completely known, but evidence shows marijuana can help control chronic pain, nausea, epileptic seizures and other neuro-muscular disorders.

Vaping and E-cigs popularity among teens continues to link to other potentially dangerous drugs. It has become easy and popular to add THC to vaping devices. The temptation to use illegal street blends can be dangerous and deadly. Sadly, menthol flavors are being used to attract younger kids to their use. This year alone saw a 78% increase in e-cig use by high schoolers. All of these introduce foreign substances and particles into the lungs and pharynx, while drying tissues in the mouth and increasing the acidity of saliva. Parents need to warn their kids at an early age.

Some experts are now claiming that vaping or E-cigs are as dangerous, if not more dangerous than smoking. The problem is the average person thinks it is safe, and the sweet flavor is drawing girls to use it. It is estimated one in five high school students may now be using these products. Many who combine high energy drinks with vaping have much higher rates of tooth decay. Sugars and flavors like

like menthol are baiting young people into a system that can easily be abused with unknown formulas, toxins, addictive agents and allergens.

From 2017 to 2018 e-cigarette use increased by 78% among high school students and 48% among middle school students. Propylene glycol, the main carrier ingredient, breaks down into acids and propioaldehyde, which are destructive to tooth enamel and soft tissue. Other potentially dangerous ingredients are vegetable glycerin and associated flavorings which add sweetness to the oral cavity allowing bacteria to decalcify tooth enamel. The greatest danger, however, is the addition of unlabeled drugs and impurities that can be added on the street. These street versions have caused mysterious and deadly lung failures among teenagers.

A third commonly used chemical is nicotine which is usually used in lower concentration than tobacco products. However, a significant amount is introduced into the bloodstream. This is because people puff up to 300-400 puffs which is equal to the smoking of two to three packs of cigarettes. A normal smoker puffs less on a cigarette to avoid the quick burn off. Research indicates that nicotine decreases blood flow in gingival tissue and as a result decreases connective tissue healing, leading to a higher rate of periodontal disease and eventual tooth loss.

This destruction is heightened by the effect of cigarette smoke on tissue. The resulting dryness will destroy the protective biofilm and increase acidity in the reduced saliva. Nicotine will also decrease the immune response in the body. The result can be tooth loss, bad breath, and possibly oral cancer. Just as a bad diet can creep up on a person and cause serious consequences, a bad habit like this can over time lead to very serious problems. The mouth is key to breaking the cycle of disease and addiction. With a spirit of encouragement and good tools we can help a lot of people. This is one important reason why Dr. Hofmann wrote this informative book. Help him spread the message.

CHAPTER NINETEEN
Faith, Hope, Love, & Science

The Amazing Adventure with MAYO CLINIC:

Narrated by Dr. Hofmann: A group of Mayo Clinic doctors and I were commissioned by The Summer Institute of Linguistics (SIL) to go into what had been a dangerous area of northern Guatemala called the "IXIL Triangle." The American Ambassador had been killed in Guatemala City by a rebellion which had spread from southern Mexico. The government fought back, and the army led by General Rios Mott defeated the rebellion and then set out to pacify this mountainous area in the north. The army had helicopter outposts with perimeter fences on hilltops much like Viet-Nam.

On the first few trips we went in with volunteers to build homes for the widows and orphans and with other medical-dental teams. We worked in conjunction with the SIL Translators who had been ministering with the indigenous Indians for many years. These brave and dedicated missionaries were translating multiple dialects of the Indigenous Indian language into written word, at the risk of death. Our missionary leader had a bounty on his head, but it was removed by the enemy commander when he realized the missionary was the person who had used his pickup truck to help his mother bury the commander's father in the middle of the night.

The missionaries eventually did pull out when the war escalated but returned when invited back in by the local tribes. Everyone soon realized how important their work was. For the first time these isolated tribes were able to preserve through written language their traditional songs, history, and culture. These tribes would now have a voice in their own governance and in their countries future policies. Many believe it was the work of these missionaries and their auxiliary teams who did more to calm and preserve order than the Guatemalan army or any other institution.

It was a great privilege to play at least a small part in this reconciliation, restoration, and renewal.

The IXIL Indians are hard-working people with strong hearts and humble demeanor. Life in the mountains is tough and they live a dignified life centered on the family. Some walked miles to see us. One child that was brought in by his mother had two abscessed front central incisors. He was about 4 years old, yet he did not budge as I injected the swollen areas to extract the infected primary teeth. He had tears, but he did not cry out despite the intense pain. Normally I would wait a week or so for antibiotics to calm a swollen tooth.

The mission outpost needed a medical team high up in the northern mountain range, an 11-hour bus trip from Guatemala City. On past missions we had been transported in yellow school buses which would rattle your bones every time they hit one of hundreds of potholes on those mountain roads. This mission, however, would be a much more complex than any in the past.

The Mayo Clinic doctors needed to transport surgical equipment and so two Canadian Twin Otter bi-props were hired to fly us onto a mountain-top landing strip. From the very beginning the trip would take a turn for the dramatic and potentially disastrous. The first plane almost overran the strip after it came in from the wrong direction and had to jump a tree line before landing. Bad communications almost ended the mission. Next came the storm.

This extraordinary enclave of knolls, mountains, and fog-laden valleys with meandering streams and quaint villages was about to be hit with a gushing rainstorm. It took only one day and evening to knock out all the power lines. Our base of operations, a small concrete clinic, lost all power. The backup generator for some unknown reason failed to work. As a small family dentist, I was the low man on the totem-pole and really did feel left out of the big picture. Even the nurses received a lot more attention as they prepared the operating rooms. No one conferred with me nor paid much attention to my role - until now! I was the only one who could treat patients with a flashlight, a couple of simple chairs, and an assistant.

For the next 2 days I was the only doctor helping the patients! Soon after getting the power up, a burn victim came in with a contorted hand. The plastic surgeon realized he could not operate on the contorted hand without a drill - and guess who had brought the only drill? Prior to this, I had rarely carried a drill in my dental setup since most of the work entailed extractions. We sterilized the drill and he placed the necessary pins on each finger to keep the hand open.

Then on Day 6 we were awakened at 5 AM by one of the night nurses calling for help as one child lay dying. He was 4 years old and had been operated on for a simple hernia. In this superstitious culture where the Sun god gives life, we were in danger of sabotaging future missions. As we gathered outside holding praying, a miracle happened which I will never forget. As we looked up the thick

106

clouds swirled around opening a hole through which a small plane flew out of. Our group of humbled doctors and nurses jumped up and down cheering like a bunch of excited kids.

The danger was not over, the boy had less than half a tank of an oxygen left which was estimated to last 1 hour during a flight which was more than three hours away. We finished the mission, loaded the buses, and drove the father and mother adorned in their traditional colorful tribal colors to the capital with us. When we arrived, we were celebrated with headlines in the National newspaper and a greeting from the President and his wife who promised to build a new hospital for future missions. The child was alive and recovering well by God's Grace.

The promised clinic was completed years later and we were some of the first doctors to operate in this modern facility. We were able to treat many medical and dental patients in a cleaner and safer environment. The Mayo Clinic's motto, "Faith, Hope, & Science" rings true as they continue to treat and heal thousands around the world in hospitals and clinics located at the far reaches of this planet.

CHAPTER TWENTY
<u>The Science of Sleep</u>
Saving Lives

Many people young and old are not aware that they are not sleeping well. They are sleeping in a sick state and do not know it. In some cases, the parents do not know their children are suffering. Hopefully this information and basic knowledge will teach you how to help others and yourself. This book is intended to provide the reader a groundwork for further study. Sleep Apnea is linked to a halt in breathing during the night which overworks the heart. There are two types of sleep apnea: Obstructive and Central. Obstructive happens when the throat muscles and tissue relax and obstruct the airway. Central Sleep Apnea is common in people who cannot process sodium correctly. The retention of water and sodium fills the lungs causing the person to wake up. It appears in those who have respiratory problems and may be a result of heart failure such as atrial fibrillation. Research is still being done to understand these dynamics.

These disorders can affect social behavior, attentiveness, and can eventually weaken the body and the heart. They can happen throughout the night, waking the person up multiple times. The person may wake up short of breath and by morning can feel drained of energy leading to daytime drowsiness. This is an exhausting syndrome afflicting people worldwide.

Sleep disorders like <u>Obstructive Sleep Apnea</u>, OSA, create cycles of tiredness leading to more and more stress and aggravating insomniac tendencies. Shortness of breath and interrupted breathing will happen right at the point when a person is about to fall asleep. The brain races and the mind short circuits all attempts to sleep. The next step downward is "SLEEP DEPRIVATION." The individual is now becoming more unfocused and unproductive and unable to feel normal. They may feel like they are sleeping and may even convince themselves that everything is ok, because they cannot remember well, have a lot of adrenaline flow, and are overcompensating. This overcompensation may be in the form of euphoria coming from the use of medications, alcohol, excessive snacking, or caffeine. All of these will fail and leave the person in a greater state of deprivation.

The less you sleep the less you will be healthy. The more you sleep the better the memory, at least this is what research since 1924 shows. Sleep helps to cleanse the brain of beta-amyloid proteins linked to Alzheimer disease. Lack of sleep lowers the immune system, decreases a person's alertness and ability to resist impulses, and stresses the heart. If the heart is weakened enough, the person can have heart failure. Studies link the lack of sleep to high blood pressure, strokes, cancer, skin disorders, addictive behavior, obesity, and diabetes. Other studies suggest a connection to dementia, hormonal imbalances, anti-social behavior, and suicide. To be healthy we must have good sleep. During sleep your body goes into regeneration mode, restoring and rebuilding damaged areas. While most of the body is resting your immune system launches a powerful offense to get rid of damaged cells, generate new cells, and modulate the immune process throughout your digestive tract.

One typical indicator of SLEEP APNEA IS SNORING. It is most common with the obstructive type disorder since the closed muscles and tissues will generate the chronic snoring. It is important that anyone who suspects they have sleep apnea contact a dentist or physician and begin a sleep study. They can then obtain devices like the CPAP to keep the airway open. These studies will record periods of no breathing during sleep, and then a specific treatment modality can be recommended.

Mouth breathing is another sign of sleep disorder common to both children and adults.

Sleep apnea involves breathing through the mouth which will dry out both the mouth and throat. Do you find yourself with a constant dry throat? This may be because you are breathing through the mouth during the day or while sleeping. Do you have a panic episode or stress caused by the constant abrupt loss of breath at night? If you mouth breath during the day, you may have sleep apnea. The dryness can be destructive to teeth, bone, and gum tissue. Often people with sleep apnea feel like they sleep well, yet fatigue creeps up during the day. A loss of focus, heavy breathing, and a lack of energy are early signs. Headaches can become more and more frequent as oxygen deprivation during the night takes its toll. These headaches can lead to increased irritability and to social issues mentioned earlier.

People who can take cat naps can avoid some of the symptoms and may seem to live a healthy life. However, Obstructive Sleep Apnea will slowly wear the body down and weaken a person as they get older, gain weight, or lose important times of rest and sleep. A dry mouth caused by mouth breathing will often cause increased rates of both tooth decay and periodontal disease.

Upper Airway Resistance Syndrome (UARS)) has been defined by Stanford Research as being like OSA where the soft tissue of the throat relaxes, reduces the size of the airway, and results in frequent arousals from sleep, un-refreshing sleep, and consequent daytime impairment. Like OSA it can include cognitive impairment (decreased brain function) and excessive daytime sleepiness but is not as severe. Girls who do not like to sleep on their stomach may suffer from this. Acknowledging early stages or variation may help you prevent the more severe form and warn others who may be uniformed. By getting the proper attention early, you will be able to apply the best methods to counter and correct patterns, habits, and stress. Tell your physician and dentist your symptoms and concerns.

STRESS & SLEEP APNEA: We still have a lot to learn about the long-term effects of Stress on the human body. We do know it is not good. Short term stress can strengthen the body in both the boot camp and sports camp examples. It can be used to build up mental, spiritual, and physical acuteness. However, stress which comes from mental anxiety, suffering, fear, sleeplessness, overwork, and many other sources can sneak up on us like slow fire. The initial warnings are often ignored, and our mind and body compensate trying to adapt. However, some individuals have a breaking point where the body spirals downward. A person with COPD (Congestive Obstructive Pulmonary Disease) may do just fine without supplementary oxygen until they have a series of events which initiates severe frustration or anger. Suddenly they realize they cannot breathe or even move. Fear takes hold and their problem accelerates into a full-blown panic attack which leads to confusion and possibly syncope, heart attack or stroke. Another trigger can be an allergic reaction to particles such as pollen, dust, or allergens from grass cuttings.

Another example is a patient who goes through some deep pain with a tooth and then faces a needle or root canal. More pain ensues, and their heart rate rises, sweat and saliva pour forth, and the mind goes into a state of fear and panic. This leads to many problems including shortness of breath, nausea, dizziness, chills, choking sensations, tingling of hands or feet and even allergic reactions. If this describes you, it is adrenaline taking control. You may fear returning to the dentist. This happens to both young and old and even tough athletes.

Over time, stress leads to tiredness, moodiness, and sleeplessness. And this deepens the sleep disorders. This can create a cycle downward. The result can be severe social, mental, physical, and emotional problems which in turn can lead to abuse or overuse of drugs and medications. In the process other problems can arise such as GERD, an acid reflux syndrome, or excessive grinding and dry mouth. Those with chronic sleep apnea can end up having a heart attack.

SLEEP DISORDERS in CHILDREN and TEENAGERS:

When you see a child putting their head back to sleep or using the "humpback" posture in sleep where the rear-end is raised and with the head down and to the side, you may have a child with a sleep disorder. Children with Excessive Daytime Sleepiness may be suffering from stress, pain, fear, or syndromes such as Ehlers-Danlos Syndrome (EDS). EDS is a condition which affects cartilage throughout the body, including along the airway. Stress can come from social, family, or school issues and changes in normal patterns. Sources of pain include teeth, stomach, and other nerve issues. Fear is often associated with stress but can have unique sources such as overexposure to tragedy, horror, or terror of any kind. Nightmares and night terrors can stress out children and parents alike.

Most children grow out of fear and stresses although it may continue into their teen years. Dr. Hofmann suffered from this as a child and confesses that it was God who helped him overcome. Science has shown that prayer and faith do a lot to ease fear and heal anxiety issues. There are other possible causes of OSA in children which include hypothyroidism, excessive growth due to hormones, allergies, and the deviated septum.

Notify your Pediatrician concerning sleep disorders which persist. A collapsed palate or a heavy overbite can be a sign of a restricted air passage. Dental appliances such as the Helix and the ALF appliances may help resolve sleep disorders by increasing the width of the palate which increases air volume. They also help tooth eruption. The ALF appliance utilizes the tongue as a functional force to shape a naturally wide palate. In doing this it can also help to open the bite, correct an overbite and improve facial asymmetry. Studies suggest increased air volume and arch width can do a lot to lower the risk of sleep disorders as they grow older. It may also help to stop snoring, which is not harmful, but is a sign air is not reaching the lungs efficiently.

Some other common causes of snoring are nasal congestion, respiratory infections, a deviated septum or enlarged tonsils or adenoids. Some doctors believe removing both tonsils and adenoids is a good help for children and may help both teenagers and adults. We know girls who snore probably have or will have a sleep disorder. And studies show women who snore have a higher chance

111

of stroke and cardiac arrest. Teenage sleep disorder can result in many hormonal and relationship disruptions. General health issues, including skin and mental health disorders are potential consequences. And it can create a cycle into isolation and depression. Quick intervention and monitoring are important to resolve problems and stop potential drug and suicidal behavior!

General Information & CONCLUSIONS RELATED TO SLEEP APNEA:
How should we treat Sleep Apnea? There are some doctors who advertise surgery on the soft palate and related tissue as a solution to sleep apnea. There is good evidence this is not a good long-term solution in adults as tissue tends to grow back. Here is more helpful information related to sleep disorders:

1)   We have clear evidence untreated sleep apnea raises the risk of heart attack.
2)   For many years the *CPAP* or Continuous Positive Airway Pressure device has been the standard of care for Obstructive Sleep Apnea. However, sleep studies should be done to determine if this is the right mode of treatment. Many people go through many types of CPAP devices to find the best one.
3)   Obstructive sleep apnea is characterized by cycles of closure and opening of the upper airway, leaving the person with intermittent lack of oxygen, heart stress and reduced sleep. Other health conditions which may arise from sleep disorders include high blood pressure, diabetes, weight gain, atrial fibrillation, polycystic ovarian disease, stroke, bruxism (tooth grinding), and dementia.
4)   However, studies show that some *CPAP* patients can still suffer from excessive sleepiness. Possible causes include the following: interruptions in the brain in areas controlling sleep; the leakage of air and the discomfort of the device or devices as in the case of a bite appliance; or breathing problems caused by changes in sodium levels related to a heart condition.
5)   Compliance by patients is a big issue. Do not give up if your CPAP does not work well for you. Do research and read the latest studies on both the internet and sleep study publications.

More research still needs to be done to answer many questions related to brain function, body chemistry, tissue and organ interactions, and the effect of anxiety and fear. Talk to your physician, dentist, and sleep clinician about your special needs and diagnosis. This book touches only the surface on the complex science of sleep disorders and is meant to alert you to take precautions before more serious problems arise. If you take no action you may be at a higher risk for a vehicular accident, isolation and depression, heart failure, drug addiction, or suicide.

112

CHAPTER TWENTY-ONE
Sugar Wars
High Octane Killer

Over consumption of 6-Carbon Sugars has created a world health crisis. On the other side is xylitol sugar which is so good that it is sold as "sugar free." If used instead of regular sugar it would help eliminate diabetes and colon cancer.

In the last 10 years diabetes has increased by 90% and strikes one in every 4 Americans. Diabetes compromises the health of millions of people throughout the world. High Fructose Corn Syrup or simply stated, "concentrated sugar fructose," which is found in most retail drinks and containerized foods is easily converted by the liver into fat. Excessive amounts will eventually lead to what is called "Nonalcoholic Fatty Liver Disease". This may then lead to an insulin resistant liver and type II diabetes. The danger lies in the fact High Fructose Corn Syrup or HFCS is metabolized only in the liver and is converted into fat and triglycerides easier than sucrose.

HFCS will increase your *triglycerides and bad cholesterol* both of which will increase the risk for heart disease and hardening of the arteries. Over time chronic diabetes will increase the likelihood of diabetic neuropathy which can lead to eventual loss of a limb or eye-sight, spinal cord degeneration, organ failure, or complications with healing after surgery.

The over-consumption of pure 6-carbon sugar and empty calories plays a similar role in harming cells and organs. Normally insulin produced by your pancreas removes the sugar from the blood quickly. As in the case of HFCS, a diet filled with empty carbohydrates and 6-Carbon sugars will overburden the pancreas. Those extra sugars are then Converted into FAT. If the pancreas is stressed too much the unused sugars will bind with proteins and denature them. These are called Advanced Glycation End - products or AGEs which can also be generated in foods as you cook them under high heat. This includes fried, grilled, and caramelized foods.

In the meantime, the excess fat formed from both HFCS and sucrose can play a significant role in sleep apnea and the blocking of the airway space during sleep. These 6-carbon sugars are a link between all three of the major oral health issues discussed in earlier chapters. Bad sugars feed opportunistic bacteria which if aspirated, can cause pneumonia or if allowed to destroy bone in the mouth can allow bad enzymes to leak into the blood vessels. These enzymes then attack heart tissue. Excess sugar will also feed the yeast Candida Albicans in the colon, where it can be a trigger for colon cancer. The fat formed from sugars can affect every organ including the liver resulting in fatty liver disease.

We already know about sugar's relationship to tooth decay, weight gain, the suppression of appetite, and the ever-present skin blemishes. It is estimated that 1/4 of the calories consumed by the average American is in the form of added sugars or empty carbs. We have made them part of our daily routine and national celebrations throughout the year. Hopefully this book will motivate you to end addictive habits and cut back on sugar intake. And do not forget that empty carbohydrates act as sugar. These starches are digested in the mouth and converted into a very sticky glue-like plaque that causes tooth decay. The following is a simplified explanation of the downward sugar spiral:

1. You have already eaten a triple mac-burger and you are slurping down a huge milkshake; 2. Your blood is now overloaded with sugar;

3. So the pancreas secretes insulin to keep up; 4. Since this has been repeated over and over again the cells in your tissues are overcome by too much sugar-to-fat conversion;

5. And blood continues to overload with sugar; 6. So the pancreas tries to keep up by producing more insulin; 7. Eventually the cells in tissue will stop responding altogether due to the sugar-to-fat overloading;

8. Then the pancreas produces even more insulin to get the cells to respond; 9. But now this added sugar which has moved into your blood stream cannot get into these overloaded cells since excess fat now blocks it.

If the glucose is not getting into cells you will feel hungry and the pancreas will keep producing more insulin to get rid of this sugar high. The result can be diabetes with weight gain while you still have hunger urges. This is the basic mechanism which creates insulin-resistant diabetes or class II diabetes. Like AGE's it will hurt the cells in many organs and limbs that depend on capillaries.

We discussed the danger of Advanced Glycation End-Products earlier. These protein end-products accumulate over a person's lifetime and can occur more rapidly in individuals with diabetes mellitus, renal failure or heart disease. AGE's can cause premature aging leading to many diseases such as cardio-vascular disease, Alzheimer's, Parkinson, and rheumatoid arthritis. This is because AGE's clogs capillaries in most structures including kidneys, heart, brain, limbs and eyes.

Food types that help form AGE's are fried foods, seared or grilled meats,

114

potatoes under high heat such as potato chips, and over-baked snack grains, Crème Brule', cola and chips. When glucose binds with proteins the AGE's are formed. It does matter how you cook your foods. Since AGE's accumulates, older people tend to have higher levels of AGE's and so need to be extra diligent. As our body ages our metabolism slows down, and our immune response tends to diminish. Our front-line defense comes from the kidney, pancreas and enzymes in the liver all of which can be over-burdened by these end products. A healthy regimen of good foods, low sugar and daily exercise helps prevent AGE's.

Sugar can do other bad things including throwing off the balance and use of essential minerals such as calcium. Calcium promotes a healthy brain, nerve conduction, and good oral health. Studies show sugar increases the rate of calcium excretion and will throw off the calcium-magnesium ratio and calcium-phosphorus balance our bodies need. This may play a part in osteoporosis.

Calcium is key to good nerve and brain function and problems with its metabolism area factor in schizophrenia and other mental disorders such as depression. We do know that xylitol strengthens bone and therefore helps with calcium transfer and absorption. Apparently, the calcium ion is shared among 3 hydroxy groups in what is called a tri-dentate ligand (H-C-OH)3, which allows the calcium atom to be released easily for bone repair or growth. Calcium is also very important to the health of saliva and therefore to the health of the whole mouth. Below are many other health issues generated by excessive sugar intake:

-SUGAR causes chronic diseases. Besides diabetes, the FDA connects both heart disease and behavioral problems such as Attention Deficit Disorder to high sugar consumption. If you reverse the word "desserts," then you ironically have the descriptive word "stressed." Over time it can severly stress the cells.

-SUGAR is also connected to Cancer. It can cause the pancreas and other organs to overwork and break down. The waste produced by overworked cells is often in the form of free radicals. It is believed that free radicals steal electrons from oxygen causing oxidative stress (like rust on iron) that can initiate mutations or cancers. When essential vitamins and minerals are exhausted, they cannot neutralize the oxidative effects of free radicals.

ANOTHER big problem is the overcooking of carbohydrates, and proteins that can cause caramelization or formation of acrylamides and other molecules which can increase the rate of cancer in organs such as the liver.

Countries like Argentina where pancakes, meats and other foods are cooked to a crisp have the world's highest liver cancer rates.

The sad thing is we are a society that celebrates the taste of sugar and alcohol. Sugar has become the drug of choice for many throughout the world. Most holidays celebrate with candy, chocolates, sodas and many forms of alcohol. We glorify brands like Hershey, Dunkin Donuts, Coca Cola, Godiva, Ghirardelli, Pepsi, and all the hundreds of other sugar creations.

The fact is we are seeing an increased rate of many nerve-related degenerative diseases including dementia, Alzheimer's, and Multiple Sclerosis. Related to these are many forms of arthritis and auto-immune diseases. Some scientists believe a link between all of these is excessive sucrose and fructose and the way we cook and sweeten foods. The 5-carbon sugar, xylitol, may be a good solution since, it is safer; having both a low glycemic index and an anti-yeast and anti-bacterial affect in the intestines, colon, and mouth. It builds up the bone and may have a positive effect on the brain. Above all this, it is naturally produced in our body and is stored in the mitochondria. This may be a good reason to call it "super-natural." The long-term evidence presented by research in Finland shows that it is not only safe for 5-year old kids but also for pregnant mothers and their fetus.

With our aging population and the increase in mouth drying medications we are experiencing an increase in the rate of both pneumonia, diabetes, pancreatitis, dementia, heart disease and many chronic disorders or diseases. This is despite our great technology, outstanding institutions, and highly educated population. We might solve a lot of these problems by looking into the progress being made in the form of prevention in many other countries including Finland. We can then adjust out priorities and focus on preventing disease instead of having to deal with the high and painful cost of tests, surgeries and other treatment.

We are often guilty of using our technology to generate fashion focused medicine that is worthless. Fads often use fear to drive and convince people that they have a problem that can be cured with a new gadget or concept. They also appeal to a person's curiosity and may do more harm than good. Examples are nasal flushes that can easily be misused and will remove the protective mucous layer in the nasal-sinus areas. The real solution is to quit the consumption of processed sugars and carbohydrates and consume low-sugar-and-acid, healthy foods and drink.

CHAPTER TWENTY-TWO
PANCREATIC CANCER
& *Periodontal Disease*

The American Cancer society says patients with pancreatic cancer account for 7% of all patients who die from cancer. In 2018, a total of 55,440 patients were diagnosed with pancreatic cancer. And it is estimated around 44,000 patients will die from this cancer this year. About 1 in 63 men are at risk of being diagnosed with pancreatic cancer and women have a lifetime risk of about 1 in 65. Heavy 6-carbon sugar consumption may have a connection to both periodontal disease and pancreatic cancer. It makes sense that there is a link between periodontal disease and pancreatic cancer. Both have specific enzymes and the body's immune reaction as a common denominator.

There have been other studies linking periodontal disease and pancreatic cancer. Finnish and Swedish scientists used previous studies to serve as a basis for their research. One study with 70 thousand individuals spanned a ten-year period and was published in the "International Journal of Cancer." An older study focused on the link between periodontitis and the mortality rate of pancreatic cancer. They found a connection between enzymes and the weakening of the immune system and how they activate certain cancer cells to invade healthy tissue in the body, (*Today's RDH*, September 7, 2018). The researchers believe the results showed periodontitis aided the spread of bad oral enzymes to parts of the body where it stimulated viral activity. This was a limited study, however, and conclusive verification is yet to be done. Researchers at the Karolinska Institute and the University of Helsinki plan to continue researching this link between oral bacteria and cancer.

The prestigious "British Journal of Cancer Study" reported in a new study that patients with periodontitis had an increased risk of developing pancreatic cancer and dying from the disease. These researchers wanted to investigate why and how bad bacteria related to periodontitis contributes to patients developing different types of cancer. They also decided to investigate the link between oral disease and cancer mortality on a larger scale. The results demonstrated periodontitis was connected to cancer formation on a molecular level due to *Treponema denticola*, a very common bacteria associated with the enzyme "Td-CTLP proteinase" and areas of bone loss around teeth. In simple terms the study showed cancer cells were formed under the influence of enzymes directly related to a common bacterium associated with periodontal disease of the mouth.

Another study by "Gut" in 2012 shows European adults with high antibody levels to the common periodontal disease bacterium strain, *P. gingivalis* were twice as likely to be at risk for pancreatic cancer. And a study by Harvard School of Public Health in Jan. 27, 2007, concluded with the same connection. The study showed after adjusting for age, smoking, diabetes, and the body mass index, men with periodontal disease had a 63% higher risk of developing pancreatic cancer compared to a control group. In a group of nonsmoking men, those with serious gum disease were twice as likely as those with healthy gums to develop pancreatic cancer.

A study by the American Association of Cancer Research shows that certain virulent bacteria related to periodontal disease increase the risk as high as 50% for cancer. The bacteria inhabit areas of bone loss and are responsible for endocarditis and other potential infections of joints and joint replacements. The researchers at NYU Langone Medical Center and its Cancer Center also found men and women with *P. gingivalis* had a 59% higher risk for pancreatic cancer. These studies have generated concern but apparently not enough to conclusively convince scientists.

The public should know the risk of allowing periodontal disease to progress once it is diagnosed. Many choose to keep their diseased teeth without corrective surgery. You should do whatever you can to control bad bacteria and enzymes even if it requires the extraction of teeth. The public should be cautious about putting dirty hands in their mouth, kissing pets, performing sexual acts, and ignoring good hygiene techniques.

Should institutions and the media do more to warn people making research data more apparent to the public? The question is how much research does it take to initiate action? Many elderly or incapacitated patients have seriously decayed teeth or periodontal issues. Colonies of bacteria in sticky plaques around teeth can also be inhaled into the lungs of bedridden patients causing deadly gram-negative pneumonia. This threat is so serious some specialists recommend the extraction of all the posterior teeth in these bedridden or incapacitated patients.

When Dr. Hofmann's Aunt had dementia, he noticed the staff failed on a regular basis to provide even a basic routine cleaning of her teeth. Each time he visited her he found that her back teeth were coated with the heavy plaque. The plaque often appears white and foamy. He then purchased a special 3-headed toothbrush and showed the staff how to use it. This brush will clean 3 surfaces at once and is effective for the handicapped, bedridden or those with dementia.

There is also a new battery powered Ultra-sonic Triple-Bristle toothbrush which could be even more efficient. Dipping the brush head in chlorhexidine or activated chlorine dioxide will help sterilize the bristles and prevent recontamination. Another simple method is to wash any toothbrush with soap and water and let it dry. He advises: "If you have an incapacitated relative, you or the nurses can use a xylitol mouth spray to help control the opportunistic bacteria. Gently rub the xylitol unto the tongue or inside of the lip. The xylitol controls acidic saliva and will also increase saliva flow counteracting the dry mouth effect of many medications. This should be done multiple times during the day, preferably right after meals. Keep them away from excess sugar."

In conclusion, research is suggesting pancreatic cancer is associated with certain enzymes produced by an accumulation of bad bacteria in a diseased mouth. It is therefore important to control periodontal disease and the bacteria associated with it. In the average clean mouth, we can control the number and kind of bacteria with diet, good habits, antiseptic rinses and with food-medicines like xylitol. Xylitol is good to use right after you eat a meal and at other peak levels of acidity in the mouth. The two other peak levels are usually registered right after you wake up and right before you go to bed. Also watch your diet, for a good fiber-rich diet can save you, whereas a sugar-rich diet can slowly destroy your body.

Links have also been established between periodontal disease and both heart disease and diabetes. Research shows bad bacteria along with other cells that are interacting with them produce enzymes which can enter our blood stream and cause cellular and tissue destruction. We should do everything possible to protect our mouth from these dangerous opportunistic oral bacteria.

Dr. Hofmann saw an older patient with four wisdom teeth which had chronic periodontal disease around them. The patient did not want them out since they were not causing pain! The teeth were not "hopeless," but they were useless since they did not add to the patient's ability to chew. There was bone loss and inflammation around each one. They were more difficult to clean than any other tooth and therefore, collected more food and bad bacteria. These 3rd molars will continue to attract infectious bacterial plaques and will help to increase the acidity of the saliva, all of which will affect the general health of the patient.

119

CHAPTER TWENTY-THREE
Tooth and Saliva Wars
TOOTH WARS:

The war to protect your teeth involves saliva and remineralization. If the pH in saliva is lowered by acids, the concentration of hydrogen ions becomes high. These hydrogen ions will replace the calcium ions in the enamel, forming hydrogen phosphate (phosphoric acid), which damages the enamel and creates a porous, sponge-like surface which is the first stage of tooth decay. If your saliva or the plaque that sits on the tooth remains acidic long enough the remineralization of the enamel will not occur, and the tooth will continue to lose minerals. This demineralization will eventually result in tooth decay. Fluoride, however, can protect these hydroxyapatite crystals by replacing the lost hydrogen ions with stronger fluorine ions which resist demineralization. These negative ions are found naturally in rocks and in our ground water. They are a natural result of ionization of fluorine which is one of the top 20 elements on earth. It's interaction with bone and teeth is a natural process that has gone on since the beginning of civilization.

Modern day fluoride has been shown to be effective against bacteria and helpful to teeth. Both sodium and stannous fluoride can work effectively with both phosphate and calcium to help recalcify teeth. A healthy saliva with fluoride works to replace lost hydrogen ions with stronger fluorapatite crystals. Fluoridated teeth are much stronger and more resistant to decay than non-fluoridated teeth. As Dr. Hofmann stated earlier, "Fluoride in water saved my teeth from decay during a childhood with a sugar craving."

The American Dental Association states that fluoride supplied through city water and consumed by a pregnant mother or a young growing child will protect teeth in their developmental stages. City water adds what is considered the perfect amount of fluoride ions by filtering excess amounts out. The standard is .7 mg/L (milligrams per liter) which is like drawing a one-inch line on a 23-mile highway. Dr. Hofmann agrees we should cut down on some fluoride intake, but many people need the protection since we are not yet on board the effort to use xylitol as a preventive. The fact is billions of kids have been born and raised with both natural and man-made fluoridated water without any negative effects. People point to videos that they have seen, yet no one can find any good research upon thousands done that shows that it causes cancer. It seems as if conspiracy lies are causing people to fear what is good.

Research indicates that stannous fluoride is almost twice as effective as sodium fluoride on the enamel of adult teeth. However, competing research shows that strength and potency may not be a big advantage in fighting periodontal disease. Although Sodium fluoride is weaker. it does not harm the biofilm and will therefore, maintain resistance to bad bacteria, help in remineralization, and prevent tooth decay and plaque accumulation. More studies still need to be done with evidence-based research.

Zinc phosphate in Colgate's Total SF toothpaste is effective against bad bacteria and in decreasing the acidity of saliva. It can be even more effective when combined with a chlorine dioxide mouth rinse or xylitol. Together they can maximize the ability to control bad bacteria, heighten the anti-odor power, and improve the ability to re-mineralize teeth. If you use a mouth rinse with zinc chloride or other zinc compound, it can also help.

As mentioned earlier there is an amazing new product called Silver Diamine Fluoride or SDF that halts tooth decay. It is especially useful for children's teeth since neither a needle nor drill is needed. Although it has been successfully used in many countries for over 5 years, it has not received full FDA approved for use on children here in the United States.

Some describe SDF as "zombie chemistry" since it spreads from one layer of decay to the next and one bacterium to another wiping them out. The bacteria eat each other and as they die, they pass the deadly silver "bullet" to the next one. Originally SDF was used only on baby teeth since it will turn the surface black after exposure to light. However, covering the SDF with potassium iodide stops the color change and allows a normal cosmetic filling to be placed over it. This amazing application is now used on adults to restore very difficult deep or hard to reach tooth decay. It can effectively and cheaply save a mouth with rampant tooth decay.

Silver Diamine Fluoride helps the dentist get to decay under crowns or on the backside of a tooth, killing bacteria and rescuing teeth without pain. Often the patient does not need to be numbed! The potassium iodide prevents the silver bullet from turning black. Then a white filling finishes out the cosmetic repair. This is an excellent solution for anyone with widespread root decay including the bedridden patient. It is also very effective on the mission field and in other remote areas where a drill cannot be used.

SALIVA WARS:

Saliva is incredibly important to the overall health of the mouth. As explained in earlier chapters saliva protects and maintains every aspect of both hard and soft tissues in the mouth, keeping them bathed in a mineral rich pH balanced solution. It is a very complex fluid which is often taken for granted. Throw it off balance and both decay and periodontal disease are more likely to occur.

Good saliva can provide an effective immune and anti-bacterial protection throughout the mouth. It can transform dry food into a molecular structure which enhances taste and then It binds the food into a slippery bolus that allows you to swallow. This process utilizes zinc to drive the taste sensation and cut down bad breath. As stated in "tooth wars" this is a good reason to include zinc chloride or other zinc compounds in mouth rinses or toothpaste. They along with xylitol help buffer acids and improve salivary flow. Xerostomia or dry mouth can negatively affect taste and the joy of eating. As stated earlier over 500 Pharmaceutical drugs and retail medications can cause a dry mouth.

The war to protect saliva starts with oral care using your sterile toothbrushes, careful flossing, and proper use of mouth rinses and water. You can use activated chlorine dioxide mouth rinse along with chlorhexidine on the spongy area of super-floss as will be discussed later. Activated chlorine dioxide mouth rinse and xylitol help to prevent mucositis and the effects of a dry acidic mouth. They both can decrease acidity, sensitivity, and inflammation.

If you want to drink frequent acids such as Apple Cider Vinegar, use a straw or take it in capsule form. After a meal follow it up with xylitol gum or a mint. Cut down on acidic drinks and foods, extra snacks and sugar-rich products. As suggested earlier Dr. Hofmann recommends super-soft or very soft toothbrushes to clean crowded teeth, difficult spots, or areas that are sensitive or eroded.

Lack of flow of saliva will lower its quality by increasing acidity. This will initiate a demineralization of your teeth followed by tooth decay. The quality can also be affected by the time of day, diet, age, sex, number of diseases and the type of medications taken.

Unfortunately, modern pharmacology seems to ignore our need for good saliva and taste. We produce and consume a great majority of the world's opioids, sedatives, antihistamines and psychotropic drugs, all of which cause dry mouth. Cutting back on heavy doses of these drugs and replacing them with alternative solutions will help saliva and the *microbiome* in your gut and mouth.

Another big development has been diagnosing disease and cancer through the testing of saliva. Testing saliva can tell us how many and what kind of bacteria inhabit your mouth. The CSI-like science of saliva testing to diagnose and prevent diseases can change the world of both dentistry and medicine.

Blood is limited to what it can transport since our capillaries are very small and blood clots can form in critical places like the brain. The analysis of saliva, however, looks at a variety of large cellular molecules to give doctors a better picture of what is clinically relevant about your health. It can measure your unique body chemistry and DNA profile in order to guide doctors in prescribing medications. They can compare over 305 drugs to tailor both type and dose while preventing allergic reactions. This testing is called Pharmacogenomics or PGx and it eliminates the trial and error prescriptions.

We know that specific variations in your genes affect how you metabolize and utilize medications and whether you will have an allergic reaction. Pharmacogenomics determines the right drug and when to administer the right dose. These genetic tools prevent toxic reactions that kill patients and cause health issues like leaky gut and dry mouth syndrome. They measure how well a patient can metabolize the drug. Everyone has different DNA and vary in the ability to absorb and tolerate a specific drug. Hospitals like the Mayo Clinic are using these advanced genomic techniques to monitor the metabolism and absorption of drugs to prevent deadly allergic reactions. The problem is so big that present estimates indicate that drug reactions or ADR's kill over 125,000 people per year in America alone.

Tissues in your mouth are very permeable allowing for the flow of various fluids which carry important information.

Also, proteins secreted through the salivary ducts warn doctors of many serious syndromes and diseases. Hormones, illicit drugs, and enzymes in saliva can also be tested. These tests can unearth important data which is often obscured in blood tests. Saliva testing tells a bigger story and saves lives while enhancing the quality of life for others.

New high-tech chips can quickly measure small levels of biologically active molecules found in saliva. These molecules are called biomarkers and by testing them doctors can diagnose propensity towards the following conditions: acne, high cholesterol, male pattern baldness, cancer, stress, heart problems, heart palpitations, allergies, cold body temperature, sleep problems, and problems with conceiving and absorbing calcium. Saliva testing is also being used by doctors in the emerging science of anti-aging medicine.

Micro-chips have been designed to measure the acidity of saliva and bad bacteria and their enzymes in saliva. Some of the biomarkers are associated with chronic and aggressive periodontal disease. An important one is called "C-reactive protein." Measuring it can determine the likelihood of disease in your heart and other organs. One system designed for this is titled, "the electronic taste chip." Research is showing biomarkers such as MMP-8 and MMP-9 may help us trace severe periodontal disease quickly. This may save lives and help detect disease or cancer in important organs like the pancreas.

OTHER EFFECTIVE TOOLS:

A good dental cleaning technique and nutritious food and drink are key to improving periodontal pocket health. The following technique may help you resolve difficult interproximal bone loss which regular floss or mouth rinsing will not help. "Super Floss" or Proxy Soft's, "3-n-One Floss" has three critical parts which work to clean and protect your teeth, bridges, and implants.

The floss is very inexpensive and comes in a 50 or 100 count. PART 1: Is the hard tip which allows you to push the floss under bridges, braces, and implants. PART 2: Is the strong superstructure of the floss which is used to floss like regular floss. PART 3: Is a "spongy" material that can absorb medicinal fluids like chlorhexidine to kill all kinds of bacteria and viruses. See Figure 7.

124

Like regular floss the super-floss must be used the correct way. If you only floss up and down snapping through the contact without pulling and pushing the floss against the curved tooth walls your flossing will be less effective.

Periodontal fibers around each root anchors the teeth to the bone. It is therefore important to keep them healthy. Practice flossing the correct way which means pulling the floss against the curved surface of the tooth and root, then down into the healthy gingival collar. This will massage and clean these precious fibers.

Healthy fiber will create pink gums. The reason is fiber is white, and since blood is red, inflamed or infected gums appear red and swollen. Even a quick up-and-down flossing is still helpful in removing the food stuck between teeth. When you see inflamed gums floss and brush them, then use a medicated mouth rinse such as one with stannous fluoride or a stabilized chlorine dioxide.

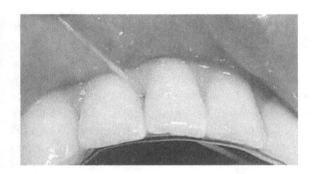

Here the plain floss is used to clean under the healthy gum collar in normal fashion & around the curve of teeth. In this case it is under a fixed retainer. Fig 8

Using the same technique above will help you kill and control bad bacteria and their spores in areas of bone loss. If you feel your mouth has been recently contaminated by an exposure to bad bacteria, you should rinse with a fast-acting spore killing mouth rinse such as activated chlorine dioxide or a potent alcohol plus essential oil rinse like Listerine Cool Mint. Although chlorhexidine also kills spores using it as a regular mouth rinse can leave a yellow stain. Brushing frequently and keeping the solution away from the front teeth helps.

Figure 7 shows how to use the spongy area of the super-floss. Like a sponge it wipes away food and bacterial in tough areas. The spongy material makes up about 1/3 of the length of the floss. When you pull this spongy part between the teeth it deposits the potent solution into the gum collar between the teeth. There are two solutions that Dr. Hofmann recommends. One is activated chlorine dioxide solution for anterior implants, ridges, and braces and the other is chlorhexidine for periodontal disease in posterior teeth, implants and bridges.

Chlorhexidine sticks to tissue, mucosa, and tooth surfaces killing both fungi and bacteria for up to 6 hours. It also kills spores and leaves a soap layer which protects the area but may create a yellowish stain. Use the solution primarily for teeth in the back of the mouth. Some dentists believe that chlorhexidine can interfere with good biofilm and the actions of fibroblasts, osteocytes, and other good cells. Dr. Hofmann, therefore, suggests using it only for deep pocket defects between teeth. If healing does not occur, you may want to consider having periodontal surgery to smooth over the bone for healing.

The best time to use chlorhexidine is at night before bed. Use with super-floss so that it will kill microbes in deep pockets and swollen gums while you sleep. If you use it as a regular mouth rinse, it can stain your front teeth. So do not use it on front teeth. Instead use chlorine dioxide or an over-the-counter mouth rinse with fluoride, essential oils and alcohol. As healing is taking place you can also use these solutions as a general mouth rinse. The fluoride rinse has the added benefit of decreasing sensitivity and the chlorine dioxide can kill microbes without hurting good cells such as fibroblasts. The biofilm with the good bacteria is then preserved. As stated earlier, remineralization of both bone and tooth requires a low acid saliva and solutions that are biocompatible with both repair cells and the regenerative process.

Dr. Ellie Philips recommends sodium fluoride instead of stannous fluoride and a good diet such as the one mentioned in this book to allow for complete healing. Her approach is to preserve the biofilm at all costs. This concept is beyond the norms of most established and popular preventive programs, and therefore, necessitates more research in a wider evidence-based scale. We need to do everything possible to defeat the ever pervasive and daunting periodontal disease that is affecting so many people.

These less powerful rinses, can motivate the growth of healthy bacteria and biofilm in the area. Your dentist may suggest one of many rinses and home care along with visits to the dental office every three to six months. Good home care and diet, however, are key to any sustainable healing and health.

126

CHAPTER TWENTY-FOUR
What is the MISSION?

A dentist should be a perfectionist who is willing to focus on a patient's unique needs. It is important to understand that everybody is different and so are teeth. This is one of the big weaknesses in how dentistry is practiced. White fillings on back molars may last many years in mouths of a petite women, but not under the pressures of the muscular male jaw. It is up to the dentist to consider all stress factors in restoring teeth. The priority should always be quality care for that patient. Often it requires wisdom to improvise a good solution. And wisdom should incorporate compassion for the patient's needs.

Knowledge alone can just puff up while love builds up. Put your knowledge to good work and the result can bring hope, compassion and of course the right solution. We should all be motivated to change bad habits and get plenty of rest and sleep so that our bodies can heal effectively for the new day ahead.

There is good evidence that nurturing a good saliva and microbiome can change the health of your mouth and body. An acidic saliva favors bad bacteria and the accumulation of hardened plaque. This is a good reason to use xylitol mints of various flavors or chew gum multiple times per day and rinse with non-acidic mouth rinses. Xylitol, fibrous foods, and chemical components in bananas, beans, onions, and garlic help to protect the gut by producing butyric acid and increasing the beneficial bacteria in the colon. A natural diet with fiber much like the classic Mediterranean diet of leafy vegetables, olive oil, garlic, fish, pomegranate juice and complex carbohydrates is also important.

If someone has a deep bony pocket, Dr. Hofmann recommends starting with the use of super-floss saturated in chlorhexidine. The chlorhexidine will kill bacteria, fungi, and spores. This is explained in the previous chapter. It helps to practice a daily oral care and see your dentist every 3-6 months for follow-up exams, at which time they can determine what other treatment is necessary.

Seek out products with zinc such as zinc chloride mouth rinses and zinc phosphate toothpastes. Xylitol is a great additive in toothpaste, drink, or food. Instead of using table sugar or other sugar substitutes use xylitol. And be aware that some companies mix erythritol with xylitol. This can create reactions such as diarrhea. The overall purpose of modern medicine should be to keep the patient healthy and decrease the need for drugs and medical intervention.

Good science should educate patients on the best methods to protect teeth, gums, and everything related to the mouth. Many in alternative medicine love to attack pharmaceutical companies for their profit motive. Yet many holistic products and concepts sold to us lack long-term testing and do not have warnings concerning both dose and allergens. Big Pharma does give precise contra-indications for use of its drugs. Improvements are needed however, as ADR's or Adverse Drug Reactions kill thousands each month. The science of pharmacogenomics is the answer. Using this simple saliva test to measure drug compatibility can save countless lives now and in the future.

Madison Avenue media-type medicine is moving us away from the good sense of Rockwell's healthy dinner table to what seems like draconian concepts of flushing, injecting, blowing, and scrubbing. Marketing and packaging have taken over. Good health should not require drugs that cause major health issues. The healthcare industry should refocus on naturally proven formulas with xylitol and products that do no harm like well-designed super-soft toothbrushes and the zinc formulated toothpastes.

Sadly, only non-xylitol sugars and sweeteners can be found in our big grocery chains. Why is this true? Why is it taking so long for xylitol to impact the entire field of healthcare? It seems that both Big Pharma, the sugar cartel and the retail medication industry are trying to edge out this natural healing food molecule. The fact that xylitol is stored in the mitochondria of our cells should be convincing enough. In the same structure are both mitochondrial DNA and RNA which have a 5-carbon sugar called "ribose" at their core. Is the 5-carbon xylitol being used to repair these and other structures or to protect cells from invasion? New research indicates xylitol does repair tooth enamel and bone by adding calcium to the matrix. It also aids in the healing of chronic infections. We need more research.

What is your mission in life? Is it to keep healthy while helping others? We cannot force people to change, but we can help them see and experience the need for good preventive healthcare. Prevention trumps having to treat disease. Your unique DNA has cellular needs that require a tailored diet with food medicines, exercise and preventive care for optimal function and protection. Study up on facts and questions presented in this book and do not listen to pundits that use scare tactics to drive you away from healthy safe science.

Beyond prevention you can take transformational steps of faith that will ease stress and offer hope. Dr. Hofmann had the privilege to serve on the first large Gospel missions to both Russia and Cuba. Both were exploratory relationship building missions. As one of many volunteers in missions by Sudan Interior Missions, SIL International, Christian Hope Indian Eskimo Fellowship, and SERVE, they were able to build modern dental clinics in Romania; bring both medical and dental care to the widows and orphans in war-torn Guatemala; help pastors and their congregation of persecuted indigenous Indians in both Panama and Peru; and treat toothaches among remote tribes in the Gola forest of Africa and other remote areas near and far. Amazing things happened during these missions including miracles.

Dr. Hofmann hopes to promote preventive techniques and solutions such as SDF and xylitol to remote communities and others throughout the world. It is a mind-blowing, soul-building experience to be out of one's comfort zone doing lawn chair dentistry and sharing the Good News. Failure may impede us for a time, but as Churchill once said, "Success is bounding from failure to failure with no loss of enthusiasm." Dentistry has its failures, but it can be immensely improved with increased honesty and a right heart. Why not refocus dentistry and Big Pharma with its mega dollars on ways to improve the quality of saliva and thus defeat tooth decay and gum disease? We will save people a lot of time, pain and money. Let's look to wholesome natural foods

He believes the Biblical manna from heaven probably had both 5 and 6 carbon sugars to provide both the energy and the protective medicine for those who had to quickly travel for years without the sustenance of their gardens.

If you are ever in our Dallas backyard, visit our mission at White Rock Lake on a Sunday afternoon, where Chapel Hill road and West Lawther Lane intersect. We have been located there for the last 9 years sharing the Gospel and giving away free inspirational books and lemonade. Each of us has been given purpose in life and the great adventure is discovering it, not only for the world's benefit, but also for our growth and blessing. The Guatemala mission described earlier was a disaster ready to happen, yet God transformed it into an amazing miracle. God has a plan for you, not to harm you, but to help you see and know the Truth behind His transforming and healing Gift of Salvation

> *"Trust in the Lord with all your heart and lean not on your own understanding; acknowledge Him in all that you do, & He will make your path straight. Do not be wise in your own eyes, fear the Lord and turn away from evil, this will be healing for your body and strength for your bones."* Pr.3:5-8

With good science, faith and perseverance we will change the world including your health and the health of those in the neighborhood. *Love Rejoices in TRUTH.*

REFERENCES

Chapter 1
1.   J. Ahn."Certain Oral Bacteria Associated with Increased Pancreatic Cancer Risk."
2.   American Association for Cancer Research (AACR) Annual Meeting. 2016 April.
3.   B.F. Bale, A.L. Doneen, D.J. Vigerust. "High-risk Periodontal Pathogens Contribute to Pathogenesis of Artherosclerosis." Postgraduate Medical Journal. 2016 November.

Chapter 2
X. Li, K.M. Koltveit, L. Tronstad, I. Olsen. "Systemic Diseases Caused by Oral Infection." Clinical Microbiology Reviews. 2000 October; 13(4): 547-558.

Chapter 3
1.   B.S. Bohaty, Clin Cosmet Investig Dent. 2013; 5: 33– 42. Published online 2013 May 15, Posterior Composite Restoration Update: focus on factors influencing form and function.
2.   Dersot JM, Giovannoli JL. J Parodontol. 1989 May;8(2):187-94 Posterior bite collapse.
3.   Dentaleconomics.com/articles-what-causes-changes-in- occlusion.html, Jul 15, 2013
4.   M Rebibo-2009- Cited by 22 articles Vertical dimension of occlusion - ACOSY-FC Formation Sleep admin | Jun 21, 2017 | News, Yes, you can die from sleep apnea– Carrie Fisher did.
5.   www health and nurses' role in assessing… Apr 29, 2009 - Dental plaque – a biofilm composed of microorganisms.
6.   www.Mayoclinic.org/diseases-conditions/obstructive-sleep-apnea/diagnosis-treatment
7.   www.Contagionlive.com/news/dental-plaque-may-provide-a-pathway-to-pneumonia -in-ventilated-patients, May 13,2017, Saloman MS.
8.   https://www.sleepapnea.org/learn/sleep-apnea-information-clinicians

Chapter 4
1.   K.K. Makinen, C.A. Bennett, P.P. Hujoel, P.J. Isokangas,
K.P. Isotupa, H.R. Pape Jr.,P.L. Makinen. "Xylitol Chewing Gums and Caries Rates: a 40-month Cohort Study." Journal of Dental Research. 1995 December; 74(12): 1904- 13.
2.   Nobbs A, Lamont R, Jenkinson H, Microbio Mol Biol Rev. 2009 Sep, 73(3): 407-450 Streptococcus Adherence and Colonization. With Very Good Illustrations
3.   YO Crystal - 2016, ncbi.nlm.nih.gov/pmc/articles/PMC5347149/Silver Diamine Fluoride Treatment Considerations in Children's Caries ...

Chapter 8
1.   H.J. Keene and I.L. Shklair. "Relationship of Streptococcus mutans Carrier

Status to the Development of Carious Lesions in Initially Caries Free Recruits." Journal of Dental Research. 1974; 53: 1295.

2. A. Azarpazhooh, H.P. Lawrence, P.S. Shah. "Xylitol for Preventing Acute Otitis Media in

3. Children up to 12 years of Age." Cochrane Database, Systematic Review. 2016 August

4. Pope-Parker, A. WJS. 2019. March 24usa, Beware of Brushing Teeth Too Long or Too Vigorously

5. Uhari M, Tapiainen T, Kontiokari T, Vaccine 2000, Dec 8,19 Suppl 1:S144-7, Xylitol in preventing acute otitis media.

6. Uhari M, Koskela M, Kontiokari T, Antimicrobial Agents and Chemotherapy, Aug 1995, p. 1820-23, The Effect of Xylitol on Growth of Nasopharyngeal Bacteria in Vitro.

Chapter 9

1. M.R. Frazelle, C.L. Munro. "Toothbrush Contamination: A Review of the Literature." Nursing Research and Practice. 2012; 2012: 420-630.

2. A. Mehta, P.S. Sequeira, G. Bhat. "Bacterial Contamination and Decontamination of Toothbrushes After Use." New York State Dental Journal. 2007 April; 73(3): 20-2.

Chapter 10

www.akamaibasics.com/blogs/learn-more/the-superpowers- of-clove-for-healthy-gums

Chapter 11

1. S. Louis. "Feeling Guilty About Not Flossing? Maybe there's no Need." New York Times Associated Press News Article. August 2, 2016.

Chapter 13

1. www.cancer.gov/about-cancer/causes- prevention/risk/diet/acrylamide-fact-sheet

Chapter 15

1. W.V. Giannobli, T.M. Braun, A.K. Capli, L. Doucette-Stamm,

G.W. Duff, K.S. Kornman. "Patient Stratification for Preventive Care in Dentistry." Journal of Dental Research. 2013 August; 92(8): 694-701.

Chapter 16

1. Harper DS, Mueller LJ, Fine JB, Gordon J, Laster LL - Fairleigh-Dickinson University, Oral Health Research Center, Hackensack, NJ.J Periodontol 1990 Jun;61(6):352-8 Clinical efficacy of a dentifrice and oral rinse containing sanguinaria extract and zinc chloride during 6 months of use.

2. Kazmierczak M, Mather M, Ciancio S, Fischman S, Cancro L. Clin Prev Dent 1990 Apr-May; 12(1):13-7 Clinical evaluation of anticalculus dentifrices.

3. Fitzgerald AS, Hess JT, Kaplan JW, Pelen J, Dardenne F, - Department of Internal Medicine,Wayne State University School of Medicine, Detroit, MI.Biofactors 2000;12 (1-4):65- 70 Zinc deficiency in elderly patients. Zinc is needed for growth & development,

4. Komai M, Goto T, Suzuki H, Takeda T, Furukawa Y. Div.of Life Science, Grad. Sch.of Agricultural Science, Tohoku U, Sendai, Japan. mkomai@biochem.tohoku.ac.jp. Zinc deficiency and taste dysfunction; contribution of carbonic anhydrase, a zincmetalloenzyme, to normal taste sensation.

5. Reyes E, Martin J, Moncada G, Neira M, Palma P, Gordan V, Oyarzo JF, Yevenes I.J Appl Oral Sci. 2014 Jun;22(3):235-40. Caries-free subjects have high levels of urease and Arginine deaminase synthesis

Chapter 17

Bowden M, INSURANCE, June 9, 2017, "Five dental scams that can put the bite on you."

Chapter 18

1. MoorePA, Hersh EV, Principles of pain management in dentistry. The ADA Practical Guide to

2. Substance Use Disorders and Safe Prescribing, Hoboken,NJ: John Wiley &Sons; 2015:31-45

3. McAllister-Sistilli CG1, Caggiula AR, Knopf S, Rose CA, Miller AL,Donny EC. Psychoneuro-. endocrinology 1988Feb;23(2): 175-87.the Effects of Nicotine on the Immune System.

Chapter 21

1. Rouse, Jeffrey DDS.9/18/2018, Southwest Dental Conference, Integrating Sleep Prosthodontics into a Restorative practice.

The Bruxism Triad, Sleep bruxism, sleep disturbance, and sleep-related GERD, Restorative Periodontics

Chapter 23

1. Fitzpatrick S, J. Kats. "The association between Periodontal Disease and Cancer: a Review of the Literature" Journal of Dentistry 2010 July-December; 1(1): 40-42. 2010 February; 38(2): 83-95.

2. Lopez L, P.C. Smith, J. Gutierrez. "Higher Risk of Preterm Birth and Low Birth Weight in Women with Periodontal Disease." Journal of Dental Research. 2002; 81(1): 58-63.

3. Griffin T, DMD, (letswinpc.org. (05/26/2017) Periodontal disease &Pancreatic Cancer.

4. Preshaw P. Alba A, Herrera D, S. Jepsen, A. Konstantinidis,

K. Makrilakis R. Taylor.7 "Periodontitis and Diabetes: A Two-Way Relationship." Diabetologia. 2012 Jan.55(1): 21-31

Chapter 24

1. Cooper, Alisa, Xerostomia: Help Patients Cope; Have Hope. Int J Dent & Oral Heal. 4:9, 160-163

2. D'Amario M, Barone A, Marzo G, Giannoni M. Caries-risk assessment: the role of salivary tests.

3. Harper DS, Mueller LJ, Fine JB, Gordon J, Laster LL. - Fairleigh-Dickinson U, Oral Health Res. Center, Hackensack, NJ. J Periodontal 1990 Jun;61(6):352-8 Clinical efficacy of a dentifrice and oral rinse containing sanguinaria extract and zinc chloride

during 6 months of use.

4. Kazmierczak M, Mather M, Ciancio S, Fischman S, Cancro L. Clin Prev Dent 1990 Apr-May;12(1):13-7 Clinical evaluation of anticalculus dentifrices.

5. Nordqvist, C. (2018, January 2). Everything You Need to Know About Dry Mouth. From https://www.medicalnewstoday.com/articles/187640.php Rev. by U.of Illinois-Chicago, Sch. of Medicine 6 Rius, J. M., Llobet, L. B., Soler, E. L., & Farre, M. (2015). Salivary Secretory Disorders, Inducing Drugs and Clinical Management. International Journal of Medical Sciences,12(10), 811-821.

6. Villa, A., Connell, C. L., & Abati, S. (2015). Diagnosis & Management of Xerostomia & Hyposalivation.

7. Ther. Clin Risk Manag,12(11), 45-51.

8. Yu OY, Mei ML, Zhao IS, Lo EC, Chu CH.Materials (Basel).2017 Oct 27;10(11).pii: E1245. doi:

9. 10.3390/ma1011124Effects of Fluoride on 2Chemical Models of Enamel Demineralization

CPSIA information can be obtained
at www.ICGtesting.com
Printed in the USA
LVHW041237230422
717037LV00022B/336